Fred Soyka knows about suffering. For twelve years he lived in Geneva, Switzerland, working for an American-based international company. A good part of that time he was physically and emotionally miserable, until a doctor suggested there was "something electrical about the air" that might be making him ill and morose.

That remark set Soyka on an odyssey of discovery to find out what science has learned about ions and their effect on humanity.

The result is this enthralling book, a volume that offers hope for easing our ills and a timely warning that we may be making our lives unbearable through modern technology.

THE ION EFFECT

How Air Electricity Rules Your Life and Health

Fred Soyka
with
Alan Edmonds

BANTAM BOOKS · TORONTO · NEW YORK · LONDON

*This low-priced Bantam Book
has been completely reset in a type face
designed for easy reading, and was printed
from new plates. It contains the complete
text of the original hard-cover edition.*
NOT ONE WORD HAS BEEN OMITTED.

RL 9, IL 8+

THE ION EFFECT

*A Bantam Book | published in association with
E. P. Dutton & Co., Inc.*

PRINTING HISTORY
E. P. Dutton edition published February 1977
Bantam edition | March 1978
2nd printing .... June 1978
3rd printing .... June 1979
4th printing

ISBN 0-553-12866-3

Bantam Books are published by Bantam Books, Inc. Its trademark, consisting of the words "Bantam Books" and the por-
trayal of a bantam, is Registered in U.S. Patent and Trademark
Office and in other countries. Marca Registrada. Bantam
Books, Inc., 666 Fifth Avenue, New York, New York 10019.

PRINTED IN THE UNITED STATES OF AMERICA

Acknowledgments

I am particularly grateful to the following who gave me so much of their time and knowledge over the years of my investigations of the elusive Ion Story. In order of my meeting them, they are:

—Professor Felix Gad Sulman, M.D., University of Jerusalem, Israel.
—Dr. ing Walter Stark, Multorgan Research Center, Lugano, Switzerland.
—Professor Albert P. Krueger, M.D., L.L.D., Emeritus Professor of Bacteriology, University of California, Berkeley.

In addition much information was kindly supplied to me by Dr. A. P. Wehner of Richland, Washington, and Mr. C. A. Laws, Oxted, England.

A great deal of assistance was rendered to me by my friends Rosemary Dudley of the Canadian Migraine Foundation, Toronto, and Professor W. Edward Mann, Professor of Sociology, York University, Toronto. Also special thanks are due to Professor Gordon R. Slemon, recent Chairman, Department of Electrical Engineering, University of Toronto and William M. Kitchen, P. Eng., of Toronto; for their advice and comments.

To my collaborator Alan Edmonds a special note of thanks.

Finally, my undying gratitude to Helen Eliat van de Velde, New York psychoanalyst, who throughout the years encouraged me to continue my search.

FRED SOYKA

Toronto
October, 1976

Contents

THE ION
EFFECT

1

"Dread in the Eye of the Beholder"

The search for information that led to this book actually began in 1970 as an attempt to prove to myself that I was neither a manic-depressive nor a hypochondriac. For ten years I had lived and worked in Geneva, and almost from the moment I moved there from New York I suffered totally inexplicable fits of anxiety, depression, physical illness, and the kind of bottomless despair that at times even led me to flirt with the idea of suicide. Neither doctors nor a psychiatrist could explain what was happening to me, but when one said vaguely that it might be "something electrical" in the air of Geneva I seized upon it as a possible explanation and spent five years traveling through Europe, the Middle East, and North America meeting scientists and amassing an awesome pile of scientific literature.

I made three discoveries. The first was that in certain places at certain times—in Geneva, in a large part of Central Europe, in southern California, alongside the Rocky Mountains and in at least a dozen other parts of the world—the air becomes sick not because of the pollution we all know about, but because of imbalances in the natural electrical charge of the air.

1

Science knows this charge as ionization, and it is vital to the creation and health of all life. When it is distorted we humans may become so physically or mentally ill that in extreme cases we may even be driven to suicide—though it is far more likely to make us tired or irritable or just generally "below par." I also found that a quarter of the population is particularly sensitive to these changes in ionization, and that I am one of these chronically ion-sensitive, or "weather sensitive," people. These discoveries alone were enough to ease my own mind: My mysterious lack of mental and physical well-being could now be explained by the fact that I was living in what, for an ion-sensitive person, must be one of the unhealthiest places on the face of the earth.

It was, however, the third discovery that led to the writing of this book. I found that man himself often makes the air just as electrically sick as nature. With this difference: in southern California, Geneva and elsewhere it is a temporary natural phenomenon, but when man makes the air sick he inflicts it upon humanity not just occasionally and briefly, but more or less constantly. In cities everywhere, in cars and trains and buses and planes, in most high-rise office buildings and apartments, man has caused nature's supply of air electricity to be so erratic that, in a sense, it can cause us humans to blow a fuse. Everyone is influenced by the ion effect, though only one in four will be troubled as seriously as I am. On the other hand, where man has tampered with ionization most people who suffer symptoms that range from inexplicable anxieties and tension, through feelings of weariness and being "out of sorts," to unnatural bursts of hyperactivity. We explain away these feelings by blaming some handy, known cause—a stressful job, perhaps, or a fight at home.

The fact is, though, that we may be putting the cart before the horse. It's just as likely that unhealthy ionization is the reason why we find that job stressful, or is the cause of that domestic rift. By distorting the electrical charge of the air through modern technology, man may be doing more to upset human physical well-being than he is by creating pollution, the bogey that haunts humanity in this last quarter of the twentieth century. You can even make the air you breathe—and thus yourself—sick by wearing the wrong clothes or by surrounding yourself with unsuitable furniture. And it's almost certainly true that it is not the much-blamed "pace of modern life" that makes most cities such exhausting places; it's the electricity—or lack of it—in the air that you breathe.

It took me five years to discover that my doctors were wrong, that I was not physically or mentally "ill." This is understandable because the most significant scientific discoveries about ions are all fairly recent, and known only to a few experts. The two most important scientific developments have taken place only in the past sixteen years, and since most of the scientists involved are underfinanced and work in isolation, often unaware of the work of others elsewhere in the world, it has taken longer than usual for these major scientific developments to become known. In fact one reason that the World Health Organization has only just begun to show an interest in the effects of air electricity on humans is the poor communications between scientists of different nationalities.

But I get ahead of myself.

In 1960, soon after I was twenty-nine, the New York–based international company for which I had worked for two years transferred me to Geneva, Switzerland. Geneva is a paradise of sorts. It sits on a narrow V-shaped plain between Lake Geneva and the point where the French and Swiss Alps converge. It has been a world center at least since the turn of the century. More international agreements have been signed in Geneva than any other place on the globe, and for that reason the old League of Nations set up many of its departments there. After the Second World War the new United Nations continued to use the city as a base for many of its activities, and scores of multinational corporations set up headquarters there for their European operations. Inevitably, there grew up a lively, sophisticated, and cosmopolitan community of which I became a part.

The first year was a young man's dream-come-true. The job was challenging and exciting; the parties almost constant, if you accepted all the invitations—and within an hour's drive was some of the best skiing country in the world. The year was marred by only one thing—I caught a cold and couldn't get rid of it. It hung over me like a small, black cloud for six months until the constant headaches and other common cold symptoms began to get me down. The cold was later to prove to have been an early warning symptom of a physical and then mental decline so serious that by mid-1961 I was beginning to lose my normal sense of well-being. The cold was followed by a bad stomach. After eating all but the plainest food I would feel nauseous. I began to avoid the social circuit, and at times even found that I began to lose my sexual drive.

Midway through my second year in Geneva I got worried enough to consult a local general practitioner. Apart from the stomach upsets I had only vague complaints about feeling below par, tense, and anxious, and so he sent me to a gastroenterologist, who diagnosed a malfunctioning gall bladder and ordered that it be removed. This, he said, would limit my gustatory pleasures but would restore my old sense of vigor and well-being.

Before the operation could take place, however, I had to make a two-week business trip to the U.S. Within three days of landing the symptoms that plagued my life in Geneva disappeared. I felt energetic and positive. I found I could once more eat nearly anything without trouble. The day before I flew back to Geneva I even dared eat a gargantuan pastrami sandwich, and still my stomach behaved itself. When I got back to Geneva I called the doctor and told him: "Look, I took my gall bladder to the States and it didn't complain. In fact, it even enjoyed it. Which means you must be wrong to want to take it out."

Two weeks later, however, I wasn't sure that I'd

been right. By then the old symptoms of bad stomach and fatigue had begun to return. Once more I was apathetic and my stomach again rejected everything but bland food. I had got into the habit of recording my feelings in my diary, using red ink to distinguish these entries from appointments and expenses. During the two weeks in the U.S. and for ten days after my return to Geneva I made no red ink entries. But then they started again: "Felt lousy"; "Tense and anxious"; "A bad night."

This time my GP sent me to another specialist, who concluded that my thyroid was underactive. He told me, in passing, that many among Geneva's "foreign" community suffered similar problems. The doctor prescribed thyroid stimulant drugs, and within days I began to feel better. Even so, on occasion I still had to take tranquilizers to steady the nerves during periods of feverish anxiety and sometimes stimulants to shake me out of fits of lassitude. At times I still needed sleeping pills to cope with insomnia. (It's important to point out here that these problems were not apparent to other people, either friends or business associates. I became a secret pill taker in much the same way that I suppose some people are secret drinkers. I felt a wreck, but made quite sure no one else suspected it.)

By 1964 I had become executive vice-president of the Swiss-based operation, responsible for overseeing part of the European operations of the New York parent company. But my troubles continued. For much of the time I felt fit, full of life and energy. But for no apparent reason there would be days on which I felt so tense and anxious that I would almost lose my ability to function. I would be beset by nameless fears and doubts that were all the more devastating because there was no explanation for them. Typically, such feelings would be accompanied by insomnia, and were often punctuated with periods of either frantic hyperactivity or total lassitude, of exhaustion and the sort of despair that was almost paralyzing. I would, for instance, find it too much trouble to make a simple phone call, or to cook a meal for myself or even put the garbage out.

So why not leave Geneva? Several of those red ink diary entries read "Get Out!" Although I did eventually leave, I was in no hurry to make such a decision. Geneva—and Europe generally—was then a paradise of sorts on a North American salary; a life that many upwardly mobile executives and businessmen back in the U.S. and in my native Canada dream about. When I felt at my worst I would swear faithfully to get out, but on those occasions I lacked the energy to do anything about it. And when the acute "attack" had passed, I would decide that things weren't so bad after all. Memory is short, and treacherous.

Anxiety is, of course, a destructive state and one of the most common afflictions of modern humanity, particularly in urban areas. Yet while it is one of the most common conditions known to psychiatrists, it remains one of the most difficult to describe. The symptoms are much the same as those suffered by someone under stress, but while you can explain stress, you cannot handily explain anxiety. Hans Selye, the world's acknowledged expert on stress, says that similar symptoms to those I suffered are the body's way of responding to stress, and that stress is an external influence, and therefore definable. If you lose your job or fight with your wife or have money problems, then these are external stresses that influence both the body and the mind, and generate depression and despair. Defining the cause of stress helps cure its symptoms. But I could find no external, rational, and therefore comforting reason for my "attacks." On the other hand, the now common condition that psychiatrists define as anxiety is irrational and unexplainable. The first man to write of it, the Danish philosopher Soren Kierkegaard, also provided the best definition: "Dread in the eye of the beholder."

That more or less describes the "attacks" that I suffered with increasing frequency and severity. And at such times tranquilizers, sleeping pills, and stimulants were of no help; by then my body had grown so used to them that they weren't very effective. Tranquilizers are, of course, called anxiolytics by the medical world, and the oldest anxiolytic known to man is alcohol. I even tried that on occasions, but drinking didn't help any either, though the temptation to seek oblivion by any means led me to have a fresh sympathy for those who have become alcoholics.

In all this there was one besetting paradox: Whenever I left Geneva on business trips, I felt fine. After a few days out of town I could eat more or less what I wanted. I slept well. I had no trouble reaching conclusions and making decisions. During an "attack" my sex drive diminished but that, too, changed when I went to Paris or London or Rome or wherever business took me. I began to look forward to such trips, assuming that the stimulus of travel offset what I had now come to describe as my "condition."

Toward the end of 1965 I went back to the doctor again, and this time he recommended a psychiatrist on the grounds that if the problem wasn't physical it simply had to be psychosomatic. So for the next two years I spent four hours a week on an analyst's couch examining my life for hidden fears, conflicts, and guilts that had waited until my midthirties to emerge from the subconscious to haunt me. When I left New York to move to Geneva I was the kind of man who was impatient with people who turned to psychiatrists to solve problems that I felt they should deal with themselves. But having experienced firsthand the kind of suicidal despair that is beyond reason and self-help, I was forced to grow more tolerant. Even so, after two years of analysis I felt no better. Those diary entries in red ink still read: "Felt terrible!" "Very ill, depressed, feel discouraged" "Sleepless night—again!" "Get out of Geneva!" "Felt like the dead, and wish I were." I would still lie awake worrying about little things—something idiotically trivial at the office, or about the future. And I worried about the fact that I was worrying.

By now I had been in Geneva for about eight

years. Life and work were, for the most part, rewarding and challenging and marred only by these frequent fits of depression and anxiety. I had lost faith in psychoanalysis, but the experience left me questioning my own emotional and psychological adjustment. Work went well enough, but despite this external evidence that I was functioning adequately by most definitions, I was troubled enough to seek medical help once more. This time I sought out Dr. Bernard Wissmer, a Geneva general practitioner whose patients were mostly foreigners. I wanted to discuss with him the possibility that part of my problem was that I was an alien in an alien land. Wissmer said that, inexplicably, many of the foreign community complained of the same or similar ills to mine: colds, fatigue, troubled stomachs, depressions, diminished sex drive. "Sometimes I think there's something electrical about the air here in Geneva," he said.

2

The Witches' Winds

The most immediate benefit of consulting Dr. Wissmer was being told that many other foreigners in Geneva suffered from the same malaise that had plagued me for years. I was not unique. For the first time, my condition began to assume the proportions of a tangible illness also suffered by others, though Wissmer did say that I appeared to suffer more from this mysterious "something electrical about the air" than most. But I was not a physical or emotional cripple, nor was I going out of my mind.

Wissmer said that many of his other foreign patients not only suffered physical problems the same as or similar to those of which I complained, but at the same time often began behaving in a manner he considered to be out of character. He said there seemed to be an unusually high incidence of broken marriages among those of the foreign community who came to him with problems like mine, and this seemed to be linked to a dropping off in the sex drive of one of the partners. For obvious reasons, men most commonly appeared to be the victims of this particular problem. They would complain that their wives no longer stimulated them. Without claiming any scientific evidence for the conclusion, Wissmer suggested this was because in the ego-sensitive area of sexual potency a man was more likely to blame his wife than himself for his lowered performance, and at the same time seek reassurance by playing around behind his wife's back. Ultimately, this usually led either to a rift in the marriage or to break-up and divorce. Women, too, would complain of feeling tense and anxious and unhappy, and believed that this ill feeling was the cause of their diminished interest in sex. In fact, said Wissmer, it seemed likely that one didn't cause the other, but rather that the anxiety and lack of sex drive were part of the same condition.

There were many other problems that Wissmer associated with his foreign patients. Excessive drinking was one. Another was tension and anxiety similar to that which I experienced. One Swedish woman, the wife of a businessman, said she had caught a cold a few days after the family moved to Geneva and was never without one for the next ten years. That apart, she would at times "find myself just not being myself— I'd swear at the children, find fault with my husband, eat too much and get fatter and fatter, and be so depressed and quarrelsome that even I couldn't stand me." And this was a woman who had happily lived in England, throughout Europe, and in the Middle East. Wissmer said that the litany of woe that he heard from his immigrant patients most commonly ended with the wail: "I just can't cope any more."

Wissmer said that patients complaining of conditions like mine seemed to come in batches. For months his practice would be much like that of any other general practitioner, and then there would be a sudden surge of patients all making the same complaints about anxiety and lassitude, sleeplessness, and being generally "off color." He had been unable to find any rational explanation for these abrupt changes in patients' spirits and medical problems.

Coincidentally, a week or so after consulting Wissmer I went to New York for a couple of months. A few days after arriving I called on Helen Eliat van de Velde, a Freudian psychoanalyst who had lived and studied throughout Europe before setting up practice in New York. Helen, who had been my neighbor in a brownstone overlooking Washington Square between 1958 and 1960, had often talked to me about the mystery of her patients' moods. She had noticed that one day most of them would be optimistic and enthusiastic, and on another day depressed and unhappy. "I can find no sane reason," she would say. "I even keep records of the weather, but it doesn't seem to matter whether the sun is shining or the rain is falling. Being weather sensitive doesn't always seem to depend on the weather."

On this visit I found Helen frantically answering two telephones that seemed to be ringing incessantly. She told me that it seemed that all her patients were having crises at the same time. The day had begun at 4 A.M. with a call from one of her patients, a woman of thirty, whose problem was classically Freudian: a love for her father and a jealousy of her mother. The night before she had fought with her mother, and her father had sided with his wife. That night the woman awoke spitting blood from a ruptured stomach ulcer. The cause, said Helen, was the woman's terror of losing her father's love.

At breakfast, Helen had been disturbed by another patient, this time a beautiful model in her mid-twenties. Apparently she had said, "I can't face the cameras today, I just can't," and then burst into tears. Her problem, said Helen, was that she had had a strict, almost Victorian upbringing but lived in a jet-set world and had suppressed guilt that expressed itself in a subliminal fear of the big, phallic lenses of the photographers.

And then there was the violinist who couldn't play that day because his hands were sweating and trembling, which always happened on what Helen called his "bad days." She didn't tell me his problem. She did say, "I tell you, there is a hurricane heading this way from the Caribbean. I know it's a fine, sunny day out but just listen . . ." She opened the window, and the dull rumble of the inevitable New York traffic jam was punctuated by yelling voices, drivers swearing at one another. "I tell you, my patients and the New York cabbies, they're like seismographs for the weather. The patients' problems become more acute, and the cabbies get ruder than ever whenever the weather is going to change."

That night the sky clouded over. It rained, and there was a high·wind. I slept badly, and sat up half the night feeling as anxious as I so often did in Geneva. Next morning, on the front page of the New York *Times,* was an account of the sudden change of course of an offshore hurricane that now threatened the southern states.

Now I had two experts in different branches of medicine—a respected doctor in Geneva and a well-known analyst in New York—talking of the mystery of their patients' changeable moods, in one case because of the weather and in the other because of "something electrical in the air" of Geneva. I seemed to be a victim of both.

A few months after my first visit to Dr. Wissmer I heard from a friend that Jack Dreyfus, Jr., the multimillionaire who founded the successful Dreyfus Fund and was at that time one of the wizards of Wall Street, was held in great respect by many medical scientists because he had discovered that some people were victims of excess body electricity. Wissmer believed there was "something electrical" about the air in Geneva; Dreyfus had proved electricity could make people ill.

I found that Dreyfus once suffered in much the same way as I did. He had written: "There was an ever present feeling of fear which varied in intensity during the day, and my mind was preoccupied with pessimistic and frequently angry thoughts. I had minor discomforts—chronic pains in the neck area and mild stomach upsets. The happiest part of the day was the time when, with the help of sleeping medicine, I was asleep." Dreyfus was puzzled because at the time his business was doing well, his personal life was happy, and there was no rational explanation for his fears, angers, and anxieties. Like me, he had tried a collection of specialists and, also like me, had tried and rejected psychiatric treatment.

One day, plugging in a vacuum cleaner, he received an electric shock and flew into a violent and uncharacteristic rage. When he calmed down he felt so much better than usual that he began to wonder whether the shock had simply triggered an explosion of excess electricity in his body, and that this eruption of temper was a sort of natural pressure release valve. In turn, this led him to wonder whether the sense of well-being after the rage was because the excess body electricity had been drained off. If so, that meant he probably had too much electricity in his system for most, if not all, of the time. His investigations showed that electricity is an integral part of all biological activity.

Dreyfus discovered that epileptics are known to have unusual electrical brain wave patterns. Doctors control these aberrant brain waves with the drug dilantin or DPH. Dreyfus began taking small doses of DPH daily. He found that it cured him. After doctors had investigated his case, he was asked to address a convention of medical scientists, and he told them that soon after taking DPH his feelings of fear, impatience, irritability, and anger "went back to what I view as normal." His physical symptoms—those neck pains and stomach upsets—disappeared. He said his mind ceased to be constantly active, to nag away at minor and largely irrelevant problems, and that he felt well again.

To me, all this sounded painfully familiar. And yet in my own case it was too simple an explanation. I realized that I felt similar symptoms to those Dreyfus described only when I was in Geneva, and that when I was away on trips or up in the mountains skiing I had no problems. In my case, therefore, it had to be Geneva that was the problem, and most probably the air in Geneva.

Perhaps because I now knew that I was not

unique, that others were similarly troubled, I began to voice my belief about the Geneva air being unhealthy. Astonishingly, friends agreed with me, and some of them knew of the age-old legends of the Foehn, the dry southerly wind that blows out of the Alps in early spring and fall and is stigmatized as a Witches' Wind. When the Foehn blows, the Swiss and the people of southern Germany blame almost everything unusual on the wind itself. Fights at home, suicides, murders, traffic accidents, even plane crashes—all are said to be part of the Foehn sickness. In Munich and many other parts of central Europe north of the Alps, surgeons even postpone operations if a Foehn is forecast.

But no one could explain *why* the wind is evil; why it blows misfortune and unhappiness as it sweeps across the plains dominated by the alpine mountains.

There are scores of so-called Witches' Winds around the world. They include the Santa Ana in California; the summer winds of the desert that stretches from northern Arizona down into Mexico (they are known in Indian mythology as the Bitter Winds); the Chinook in western Canada and the U.S.; the Sharav (or Hamsin) of the Middle East around Israel. All are infamous, perhaps the Foehn most of all.

In Munich, a good friend learned to fear the Foehn because it made it impossible for her to sleep. For years she had inexplicable but occasional bouts of sleeplessness and irritability. They seemed to have only one common factor—train whistles. As she lay awake, reading or just tossing and turning, she noticed that she could faintly hear the sound of trains. That in itself was unusual, since the tracks were miles to the south of her apartment. By a process of deduction similar to mine, she realized she slept badly only when the wind blew from the south, and that wind was the Foehn. Another friend in Munich, a British-born artist, cycles around the city all year— except when the Foehn blows. "For some reason the drivers all become either madmen or an accident looking for a place to happen," he says. "To ride my bike would be asking for trouble."

In the south of France, along the glorious blue of the Mediterranean as it washes the Cote d'Azur, I met an unhappy honeymoon couple from Montreal. The husband, a young lawyer, had arrived a few days earlier with the vigor and enthusiasm one might expect of the occasion, and within a day was squabbling with his bride. He said he felt tense and worried one moment, and exhausted the next. The Mistral—the Witches' Wind of southern France—was blowing. The couple left for less romantic surroundings four days after arriving, and later wrote to say the husband's mood had changed and they had, after all, had a wonderful time. In southern France the Mistral is infamous. Biographers say Winston Churchill chose the dates of his visits to the Mediterranean coast of France with care to avoid the wind, and Gertrude Stein hated visiting the south of France in the Mistral season since, while that ill wind blew, she was always tense and morose, snarling at her hapless companion, Alice B. Toklas.

Along the Rocky Mountains in the western U.S. and Canada, the warm, dry Chinook flows eastward out of the mountains for a few days at a time every year as winter is about to give way to spring. Since it provides relief from the bleak chill of the lingering prairie winter, it is regarded as a benign, beneficial wind. But is it? Doctors say the Chinook coincides with outbreaks of the common cold and other respiratory ills (though this is usually blamed on sudden temperature changes), and I know one successful industrialist who after a decade or so found the Chinook made him feel so ill—he, too, suffered anxieties as well as colds—that he now carefully schedules his holidays so that he escapes the area each spring.

In southern California, the hot, dry Santa Ana wind streams out of the coastal mountains across the plain where cities sprawl into one another from north of Los Angeles and Hollywood down to San Diego in the south. The belief that it causes murders and suicides and violence is so widespread that the Santa Ana is even used as the explanation for crimes in the private eye stories of Raymond Chandler and Ross MacDonald. In the Middle East some courts even permit the fact that the Sharav was blowing at the time a crime was committed to be entered as a plea of mitigation, while in parts of Switzerland and Italy judges are often known to be lenient if the local Witches' Wind was blowing at the time certain offenses were committed. In the Arizona desert, local Indian mythology tells of people who are susceptible to what they call the Wind Sickness.

These Indians and the others mentioned here are probably among the quarter or more of the human race who are "weather sensitive"—human barometers whose minds and bodies are thrown violently out of balance in response to changes in the weather. Here I am not talking of those who suffer acutely from extremes of heat or cold, since their problems begin when the hot or cold weather front has actually arrived. We call people weather sensitive when they are so affected that they can even predict a weather change. They may develop a violent headache or begin to feel depressed and out of sorts or even overactive and hyper. An old injury or wound may begin to ache. Such people are almost certainly affected by the advance guard of distorted air electricity that heralds a new weather front. The old salt who announces that "it's going to rain; I feel it in my bones" is often right. As we age, our bodies may become less able to cope with such changes in the environment, and experience may also make us aware that the ache or the headache or whatever usually occurs before a thunderstorm.

It was not until now, however, that this kind of folk wisdom had a scientific explanation. Even though I later found that most of my problems in Geneva were similar to those of people known by their doctors to be weather sensitive, it wasn't until 1971 that I finally made the connection between my "Geneva condition" and air electricity. At the same time I found that not only weather sensitive people are affected by electricity in the air. A large slice of humanity is influenced, most noticeably in the path of the Sharav in

Israel; the Foehn in Switzerland, southern Germany, and Austria; the Mistral in France; the Sirocco in Italy; the Santa Ana in California. The acutely weather sensitive may go to doctors with an encyclopedic collection of physical and mental ills ranging from swollen feet to serious psychiatric problems. Others are equally affected, and, without a sane explanation for their feelings, are driven to extraordinary acts. In all these areas, both the suicide rate and number of attempted suicides soar when the Witches' Winds blow, and traffic accidents become almost epidemic. Most people, of course, just feel low and out of sorts. Admittedly they blame their feelings on the weather—but on the fact that it may be cloudy, humid, or a day of dreary drizzle. It's when there is no *visual* change in the weather, as is often the case with the Witches' Winds, that these seemingly inexplicable feelings are most damaging.

In a similar way everyone may be equally a victim of the man-made twentieth-century Witches' Winds that we create in cities, in modern buildings with central heating and air conditioning, and in cars and other forms of transportation.

It is not the weather itself to which people are sensitive so much as those electrically charged molecules of air called ions—that "something electrical about the air."

3

The Critical Ion Balance

When I began investigating the ion effect, I soon found
that I was hardly a pioneer. In fact, I discovered that
so much was already known about ionization and its
effects that the astounding thing was not so much the
effect that ions have on us all, but that hardly anything had been done with the knowledge already available.

Working in isolation thousands of miles apart, the
natural philosophers—which is what we now call early
scientists—of the late eighteenth and early nineteenth
centuries all reached the conclusion that "air electricity" affected plant growth and probably all living
things. The lightning conductor was simply Benjamin
Franklin's practical application of his theories about
the importance of electrical energy. But he reached
those conclusions without knowing of the work of the
Frenchman L'Abbe Nollet who, in 1748, found that
plants placed under charged electrodes grew faster, or
of Father Gian Battista Baccaria of the University of
Turin, Italy, who in 1775 wrote: "It appears manifest
that nature makes extensive use of atmospheric electricity for promoting vegetation and besides [such elec-

18

tricity] constantly prevails when the weather is serene and certainly contributes to promote vegetation. And we have also observed that artificial electricity has the same effect."

It was not until the 1890s, however, that scientists found that this air electricity comes from charged molecules—or ions—of gas. In the 1920s science still knew little about the phenomenon, but researchers had begun to take seriously the claims of the natural philosophers who argued that air electricity was in fact a vital part of the process that creates and sustains life. Only in the past decade, however, have scientists been able to actually prove that when nature or man starts meddling with air electricity, life can become insufferable for some of us, and uncomfortable for all of us.

As is the case with all matter, the air is made up of molecules. Each molecule has a core, or nucleus, of positively charged protons surrounded by negatively charged electrons. Nature constantly seeks an equilibrium in all things, and in this case it seeks a balance in which there are as many electrons as protons so that the positive and negative charges cancel one another out. This happens in a stable, or passive, molecule of air. But while you may not be able to see a molecule, scientists can actually weigh its component parts. Since an electron is 1,800 times lighter than a proton, it is the electron that is most easily displaced—and when that happens the equilibrium is upset and a "maverick" molecule, or ion, is created.

The active electricity in the air comes from these "maverick" molecules—those that have lost or gained a negative electron so that the equilibrium is upset. If a molecule loses an electron it becomes positively charged, while if that displaced electron attaches itself to a normal molecule, that molecule becomes negatively charged. In what nature considers "ideal" environments for living things—that is relatively clean air over open country—the energy needed to displace electrons and so create charged molecules comes mostly from the minute quantities of radioactive substances that are present in the soil and rocks everywhere, and from the rays of the sun.

Ions come in three sizes: large, medium, and small. It is the small ions that are absorbed by living matter, from plant leaves to human tissue. It's these small ions we're talking about here; the larger ones have no apparent effect on living organisms.

Because the earth itself is negatively charged it tends to repel the negative ions, to drive them away from the area near the surface where life of all kinds exists. Similarly, it tends to act as a magnet to positive ions and draws them into this surface area. Consequently, there are usually more positive ions than negative ions even on a glorious summer's day in the country. The accepted scientific wisdom is that while there are somewhere between 1,000 and 2,000 ions in every cubic centimeter of air over open land, the usual ratio is five positive to four negative. It is in this ion ratio, or balance, that life evolved. Scientists at the University of California grew barley, oats, lettuce, and peas with a total of only sixty positive ions and negative ions and found that growth was stunted and the plants were diseased. The same experiment in air with more than double the natural number of ions produced accelerated growth. In Russia, scientists tried to raise small animals—mice, rats, guinea pigs, rabbits—in air with no ions in it at all. They all died within days.

The fact that in air with a low ion count plants wither and animals die underlines the importance of ion count in the process of creation, since plants are the source of all life-giving energy on earth. Apart from their significance as the start of all food chains, plants live on nitrogen, which is a waste product of all animal life, and they create oxygen, which we all must have to live. The process by which plants do this, photosynthesis, could not take place without ions in the atmosphere. James B. Beal, formerly of the National Aeronautic and Space Administration, who came across the ion problem while studying the kind of environment needed in space capsules, has written: "The human race was developed in ionized air. Nature used the ions in developing our biological processes." In Japan, Russia, Israel, Brazil, and throughout Europe scientists have proved that it's not only unhealthy for plants and mice when the natural ion count is upset, it's just as damaging to human physical and mental well-being. That natural ratio, or "balance," of five positive ions (or pos-ions as I will call them) to four negative ions (neg-ions) is another example of nature struggling to achieve equilibrium: Ions of both charges are presumably vital to normal life, and the ratio seems to be as important as the total number of ions in the air.

You can upset the balance one way and do harm, yet if you do it the other way it seems to do nothing but good. By now there are around 5,000 scientific documents in a score or more languages reporting experiments with ionization, and all support the conclusion that, generally speaking, an overdose of pos-ions is bad for you while an overload of neg-ions seems to be beneficial.

Although humanity has done the most to produce unhealthy ion levels, nature itself often produces overdoses of both kinds of ion. Pos-ions can be produced by various kinds of friction: between air masses, between layers of wind, between the air and the ground over which it is blowing, between the air and sand or dirt particles swept up by the wind, between the weather fronts that march endlessly across the face of the globe. Friction tends to knock off the negative electrons and produce an overdose of positive ions. On a dusty or humid day this overdose may be massive because the neg-ions promptly attach themselves to particles of dust, pollution, or moisture and lose their charge.

The weather changes when one atmospheric front is shoved out of the way by another. If there are rain clouds, the rubbing of the new front against the old, and of cloud against cloud, commonly causes thunderstorms because the rubbing sets up a positive charge that flashes to the negatively charged earth as lightning, destroying the overdose of positive ions as it does so.

But the electrical disturbance moves faster than the weather front, so that in the hours or days before the arrival of an electrical storm the air is overloaded with positive ions. It is these that cause animals to be restive and insects to erupt suddenly with an explosion of energy and become a plague instead of just a nuisance. It is part of the lore of humanity everywhere that if livestock is restless and the bugs begin to bite more than usual, then a storm is probably on the way. Scientists studying the incidence of insect activity in laboratories have now provided the scientific reason why: Pos-ion overdoses affect the body chemistry of all creatures.

When the storm has passed, however, the air is fresh and clean and invigorating. Most of us feel vigorous and refreshed and at peace with the newly washed world. The reason seems self-evident: The storm has passed. But again, scientists have demonstrated that the storm's passage has cleared the air of positive ions. What is left in the wake of the storm is a gloriously tranquilizing overdose of negative ions that eases tension and pressures and leaves us full of energy.

Not all moving weather fronts bring storms with them, however; they may simply bring slightly higher or lower temperatures, changes in air pressure, or fewer or more clouds. Even so, there is usually an advance guard of air carrying a heavy positive charge, and as a result animal and insect activity still increases, although there is no visible reason why. It is one of the paradoxes of the ion effect that while a pos-ion overdose is damaging, a brief dose may at first produce a short spell of euphoria, hyperactivity, or a sense of suppressed excitement. Other life forms—the insects, for instance—seem to feel this more intensely than humans, and weather- or ion-sensitive people seem more likely to feel depressed or tense and anxious. In both cases the feelings are apparently inexplicable since we are feeling the effects of something we cannot perceive with any of the five senses—we can't hear or smell or see anything, nor can we taste or touch it. In the case of ion-sensitive people, the feelings of anxiety and depression are the more disturbing because they are often a contradiction of the glorious day all around.

Electrical energy created by friction is also the problem with the Witches' Winds. The two most studied of these—the Foehn of central Europe and the Sharav (or Hamsin, as the Arabs call it) of the Middle East—are typical of such winds. These Witches' Winds can be, and usually are, winds in the common definition, or they can be "falling winds" created when a body of air from the upper layers of the atmosphere falls down toward the surface of the earth. Whether traveling across the surface of the earth or falling from on high, there is friction with the surrounding air. In the Foehn, which blows from the southeast and follows the contours of the Alps of Switzerland, France, and Austria, the wind both falls and blows, and its upper layers, having farther to travel, rub against the lower layers. With the Sharav, which also begins life as a falling wind, there is the added friction caused by the thousands of tons of dust and sand that the wind picks up as it crosses the arid, trackless deserts of the Middle East. Both the Foehn and the Sharav are warm, dry winds so that there is insufficient moisture in them to readily conduct the electricity they carry to earth. Neg-ions attach themselves to the sand and dust and lose their charge. Without moisture in the air the positive ions are not conducted to earth, and thus the longer the wind blows the greater the build-up of positive ions. In the case of both winds the effect is much the same as it is with a thunderstorm: Electrical disturbances arrive hours or even days ahead of the wind itself. In Jerusalem, Sharav victims report their greatest mental and physical anguish in the two days prior to the arrival of the Sharav itself. In parts of Foehn-afflicted southern Germany hospitals cancel operations a day or so before the predicted Foehn arrives. At the same time the traffic accident rate rises by more than 50 percent and the number of suicides and attempted suicides soars to epidemic proportions.

There are also circumstances in nature that create

overdoses of the neg-ions that are good for you. In certain hill and mountain areas, for instance, a combination of the sun's rays, cleaner air, and rock strata that are more radioactive than most of the earth's surface can produce high concentrations of both kinds of ions, with the balance swinging heavily in favor of negative ions. In part this is because in the mountains there is less dust in the air to consume the neg-ions. It is no coincidence that throughout history mankind has gone to hilly areas to rest and recuperate, particularly from respiratory diseases.

The energy in moving water also generates a lot of neg-ions since, as water breaks up, the positive charge remains with the larger drop and the negative charge flies free with the fine spray, forming neg-ions. By the seashore, where waves bounce on beaches or hiss and sputter against rocks, there are always more neg-ions than pos-ions. Waterfalls, too, are surrounded by a beneficial load of neg-ions created by the same process. The easily measurable negative charge in the air of Yosemite Valley is said by physicists from Stanford Research Institute to be due to the famous waterfall there. At one Russian spa scientists have found a total ion count of 100,000 per cubic centimeter, with neg-ions being in the majority. A few hundred yards away the count drops abruptly to a normal 1,000 to 2,000 ions per cubic centimeter. No one has yet taken measurements near Niagara Falls, but the fact that it is the most stupendous neg-ion generator in the world and that neg-ions produce a sense of well-being may be the reason why Niagara has been a honeymooners' paradise for almost as long as the area has been accessible. The honeymoon of the young couple I met in the Cote d'Azur was clearly disrupted by the Mistral, the Witches' Wind that scours a large part of France south of Lyon. It had begun to blow the day before they arrived. And all this clearly explains why a shower is refreshing under any circumstances; the man-made mini-waterfalls produce a massive overdose of neg-ions.

In Geneva, I had a neighbor who suffered as I did from tension and anxiety during the Foehn in addition to migraine headaches, an affliction I was spared. After several years of pill taking, she found her own solution to the most acute attacks. In the center of Geneva the lake narrows and flows over a small waterfall to become the River Rhone. At that point there is a bridge for pedestrians to cross the river. Each day during the Foehn she would at some point go and spend between thirty minutes and an hour leaning over the railings, apparently just an idle passer-by who had become absorbed by the dancing waterfall and the swirl and eddy of the water. In fact, she explained, "I go there just to breathe. It makes me feel better for hours."

It's obvious that nature is not consistent in its ion production. Mankind has long known that the soil in some places is better for growing certain plants than others. Historic farming practice has long enshrined this knowledge. Yet scientists studying ionization have only recently provided a possible explanation: Some land generates more ions, probably because of a higher content of radioactive materials, than is normal.

In the 1960s one U.S. Department of Agriculture scientist grew seedlings in ion-enriched air and produced cucumbers eighteen inches longer than normal. E. L. Sharp, of the Department of Botany and Microbiology at Montana State University, reported in 1971 that the spores of the wheat rust fungus, which destroys prairie grain crops, did not germinate—that is, they were in a state of stasis or "living death"—in extreme pollution, when the ion count was low. The spores revived, however, when the neg-ion count went up. University of California researchers working with barley, oats, lettuce, and peas found that high densities of either pos-ions or neg-ions produced significantly bigger and healthier plants.

But when man upsets the ion balance he does so totally and permanently. Pollution, for instance, is not seasonal. Besides which, man builds cities and covers the land with asphalt and concrete. That prevents the normal generation of ions, so there would be fewer ions in an urban area anyway. But then man creates pollution and that makes things worse. Neg-ions are more active than pos-ions—scientists describe them as "zig-zagging around at great speed"—and more readily attach themselves to submicroscopic particles of pollution. These newly charged particles cluster together to become large ions that have no apparent effect on living things, and eventually fall to the ground as dust. Thus the bigger the city the lower the total ion count, and the greater the pollution the greater the imbalance in the ratio of pos-ions to neg-ions, leaving a preponderance of the more harmful pos-ions. Buildings with air conditioning and hot air central heating systems suck in this already unbalanced air and make things worse.

Ions don't live long anyway; the charged "maverick" molecules either revert to their stable, or passive, structure, or are drawn to dust and moisture particles to become large ions that have no apparent effect on living matter. In nature ionization is a constant process; in man-made environments that process is hamstrung. Man distorts that natural ionization which former NASA scientist James Beal described as having been used by nature "in developing our biological processes." In fact, there are 27 *thousand trillion* stable, or passive, molecules of air—that as the University of California's Dr. Albert P. Krueger says, the world of science may be forgiven for having failed for so long to take ions seriously as a major influence on life.

The findings of Dr. Krueger, and of Dr. Felix Sulman, a medical scientist who has worked in Jerusalem during the past decade, have done more than anything else to make the world of science look again at the theories of Ben Franklin and his fellow natural philosophers. As Sulman said when we met in Jerusalem, each and every human being on earth breathes 2,500 gallons of air every 24 hours. We are constantly bathed in that air, whether it has a normal ion ratio or not. It seems self-evident that, since human beings and all living creatures are known to function largely because of bioelectricity, the electrical nature of the air must have some effect on all life forms. However, both scientists and the medical establishment have steadily refused for most of this century to accept the notion that ions have any biological effect. That is, they have refused to accept the idea that ions could have any influence on our bodies and our minds. The world is still full of skeptics, but they are fewer in number since America's Dr. Krueger and Israel's Dr. Sulman began their research.

4

Two Giants
of Ion Research

Dr. Felix Gad Sulman is a bespectacled gnome of a
man with seemingly endless energy and an eclectic
intellect that enables him to speak with disconcerting
expertise on subjects as varied as Etruscan history and
the social significance of the plot in whatever the current melodrama series on Israeli television happens to
be. He talks a lot with infectious enthusiasm and,
along with the mannerism of peering over his horn-
rimmed spectacles as he waits impatiently for an answer to questions, he has a habit of assuming that you
know as much as he does about whatever subject is
under discussion. It's a characteristic I've noticed in
many modest men of considerable achievement; they
don't consider themselves or their knowledge remarkable, and they assume you know as much as they do.

Sulman is a German-educated doctor and veteri-
narian who emigrated to Israel in 1932, when the
Promised Land was a protectorate administered by the
British. I first met him at the Hebrew University in
Jerusalem, where he is head of the Department of

Applied Pharmacology. I had flown there from Geneva to ask whether, though I was not an Israeli, he would treat what I had come to call my "Foehn sickness." I explained that I had all the symptoms of the people he was treating for problems related to the Sharav. I spent two weeks in Jerusalem, being examined on most days and on others awaiting the results of laboratory tests. He and his small army of assistants finally diagnosed my problem. I was acutely sensitive to pos-ions. What I had not known was that when there are too many of these pos-ions in the air my body produces an overdose of the stress-response neurohormone serotonin in my system. The pos-ions also affected the normal functioning of my thyroid gland, though precisely how they did so was then, and still is, a mystery. However, the effects of pos-ion poisoning upset my body chemistry and caused the depressions, despair, anxiety, sleeplessness, and other symptoms I had come to associate with my condition. In this respect, I am part of what Dr. Sulman, echoing other scientists, described as "the poor unfortunates who make up a quarter of humankind," although he pointed out that almost everyone else is affected to some extent by ion imbalances.

Dr. Sulman's work in ionization has given him international stature in the fledgling science of biometeorology—the study of the effects of weather and environment on human beings. Yet his involvement in the subject came about almost by accident in 1957, when an eager research student at the university hospital department of gynecology persuaded Dr. Sulman to join him in studying the part played by serotonin in pregnancy. Serotonin was then the newest discovery of scientists trying to answer the endless questions about how the human body works. First "found" in 1950, it is one of the more powerful of the neurohormones produced by the body, causing significant physiological changes, and has a massive effect on the nervous system as well. Like the better-known neurohormone adrenaline, it is a control mechanism produced in response to an external stress to enable our minds and bodies to cope with new circumstances.

Even now little is known about just what serotonin does or how these neurohormone control mechanisms work, but it seems likely that while adrenaline is produced in response to threats to our survival that we can detect with one of the five senses, serotonin is our body's response to threats that we can't perceive through our senses. Emotional stress, for instance, seems to produce serotonin. In his book *The Healing Mind,* Dr. Irving Oyle describes serotonin as "the ultimate downer," while norepinephrine, a relative of adrenaline, is the ultimate upper.

At the time Dr. Sulman began his studies, investigation of serotonin was a glamorous area of research because the neurohormone was newly "discovered." Dr. Sulman had not yet heard of Albert Krueger, whose laboratory work on plants and mice in California he was later to apply to human beings with such spectacular results. Nor did he know of the work on ionization already done during the previous three decades in Europe, Russia, the U.S., and Japan. Within the next twenty years, however, Dr. Sulman and his team of scientists at the School of Applied Pharmacology in Jerusalem were to produce what is so far the most compelling evidence that the ion balance is critical to the physical and emotional well-being of us all.

For centuries it has been part of humankind's accumulated wisdom that in some places and at certain times people can become out of sorts because they're "under the weather," and the awareness that "ill winds" exist is as old as human history. We know, then, *what* happens in certain weather conditions. Until Dr. Krueger and Dr. Sulman, though, we had no inkling *why* or *how*. Now we do, and that's partly why the World Health Organization and World Meteorological Organization got together two years ago to study the subject, and to try to bring certain environmental perils to the attention of architects, builders, town planners, automobile and aircraft designers, and others who create the man-made environments most of us live in.

But again I get ahead of myself. Throughout the 1920s and 1930s scientists in Europe—in Germany particularly—and in Japan and Russia had conducted experiments that led some to claim that ions had a pronounced effect on all life forms. Their conclusions were not accepted by science generally, nor by the medical profession as a body, although many individual doctors were believers. With the outbreak of the Second World War ion science was suspended as scientists who had hitherto been seeking ways to help humanity were put to work devising ways to destroy it. After the war the concept of an international scientific community freely exchanging information was, for a while, quite dead. That fact apart, the great technological advances that had come about because the western world and Japan had created the most monstrously magnificent war machines in history tended to discredit a lot of earlier science that relied on pre-War measuring techniques and equipment, which were not as sophisticated as those that existed later. The work in ionization was a major victim: The new sophistication in electronics led already skeptical scientists to disregard the earlier ion science on the grounds that the measuring techniques that had been used were suspect.

There were other reasons why American scientists, bursting with pride at their wartime achievements, did not take ion science seriously. Much of the important work in ionization had been and continued to be done in Russia. From the beginning of the Cold War in the late 1940s, any hope of an exchange of scientific information between the U.S. and the U.S.S.R. ended. It was also true that the political stance of each superpower led it to denigrate the achievements and potential of the other, so that even when the American intelligence community produced evidence that Communist bloc countries were active in the field of ionization, and that they believed it could have important economic and even military implications, U.S. scientists tended to disregard the information.

There is also a more basic difference in attitude between the scientific communities of eastern Europe and the U.S.: In Russia, Hungary, Poland, and other nations where significant discoveries were being made, the philosophy of science is generally European. That is, building on the experience of generations of people living in the same environment, science accepts certain phenomena as established fact. Scientists set out to find out *why* something happens. In the U.S. and Canada, where white people have lived for only the blink of an eyelid in terms of history, science demands the solution to a more basic problem: Find out *whether* it is true that so-and-so happens. In North America the *why* comes later. This partly explains why U.S. science did not tackle the subject of ionization in any significant way until the mid-1950s, and then it did so at the instigation of business rather than the scientific establishment.

Wesley Hicks, founder and president of the Wessex Electrical Company in California, had heard of the pre-War work on ions and knew of the common belief that positive ions were unhealthy to humans. He feared that electric heaters his company manufactured produced pos-ions: He had had complaints from customers who said the heaters gave them headaches, made asthma victims worse, and generally seemed to create "dead" or "heavy" air in the rooms in which they were used. Hicks financed research at Stanford University into the kinds of electrical circuitry that could produce pos-ions, and as a result the heaters were modified.

Hicks's curiosity was aroused, however. He had changed the heater design and the complaints had ended, but now he wanted to know *why* pos-ions caused these problems. In 1956 he posed the question to Dr. Albert P. Krueger, a microbiologist and experimental pathologist, who was then chairman of the department of bacteriology at the University of California at Berkeley, specializing in medical pathology and microbiology. Dr. Krueger is a tall man of military bearing with an impregnable, almost stately dignity that hides the intense and imaginative curiosity that all brilliant research scientists must have. When approached by Hicks he was fifty-four, a man who had reached the top of his field disconcertingly early, and had become heavily involved in administration.

Though he did not recognize it at the time, he was then looking for a fresh field to conquer; a fresh *why* to haunt his life.

When I first met Dr. Krueger in Berkeley in 1972, he described his encounter with Wesley Hicks this way: "I knew nothing about ions, in fact I'd never heard of them, so I went over to see Mr. Hicks completely naive and looked at these experiments done at Stanford. From a biological point of view they weren't very satisfactory. Well, Hicks asked me to work on ions and said that if I would it would make him and his associates very happy. We had a few more meetings and he offered me a grant to do the work, and as I had a sabbatical coming up I agreed to look at the subject for one year only."

In that year Dr. Krueger worked with bacteria of the kind that float in the air and spread diseases— mostly colds, influenza, and other respiratory ills—and found that an astonishingly small quantity of neg-ions could kill them and quickly take them out of the air so they were less likely to infect people. By then Dr. Krueger knew that before the War many scientists had claimed that ions had an effect on living things. He also knew that none of them had been able to back up their claims by showing why and how the ions did so. "By the end of that first year I was absolutely fascinated with the subject," he told me. "I felt the evidence I had found was clear proof that ions had some biological effect, and I wasn't aware that any such evidence existed elsewhere." In fact, it didn't. He promptly resigned as chairman of the department of bacteriology and set up his own two-room research laboratory in the Life Sciences building. Ions were, he felt, "a great challenge."

Dr. Krueger's reputation was enough to attract a group of some of the university's brightest young researchers, and for the next three years they conducted experiments that, in technique and equipment, could not be faulted. They experimented with large groups of mice, keeping some in air with a "natural" ion balance, and others in air starved of both neg-ions and pos-ions. Some were raised in pos-ion atmospheres, some in neg-ion atmospheres, and some with no ions at all. The mice were minutely examined when alive, and again when dead and dissected. By 1960 Dr. Krueger was ready to publish a scientific bombshell: In the prestigious *Journal of General Physiology* he and assistant Richard Smith announced their theory that an excess of pos-ions caused the overproduction of serotonin in mammals and that, initially at least, this causes hyperactivity which rapidly leads to exhaustion, anxiety and perhaps depression. They also said that an excess of neg-ions appeared to have an anxiolytic effect—that is, they are calming, able to counteract the effect of a pos-ion overdose and generally duplicate the effect of the common tranquilizer reserpine in that they reduce the amount of serotonin in the mid-brain. It was this, they said, "which apparently accounts for the tranquilizing action" of neg-ions.

Apart from the fact that their experiments were the first scientifically acceptable ones in the U.S. to demonstrate that ions do have an effect on living creatures, there was a hidden implication that in time may prove to be even more important: Neg-ions, a product of nature that have no known harmful side effects, do the same job as chemical tranquilizers that do have side effects, not all of them desirable. Since the Thalidomide disaster, the perils of the use of drugs to treat all and any illness have caused increasing concern in medical and scientific circles.

Dr. Krueger and his colleagues were to expand their experiments in the 1960s and early 1970s to include rats, rabbits, guinea pigs, insects, and plants, and the results consistently tended to support the original hypothesis that ions were, as they put it, "biologically active." But that original paper in 1960 was the most significant since it caught the imagination of other scientists throughout the world. Other investigators conducted experiments that generally supported Dr. Krueger's hypothesis. Perhaps the most exciting evidence came from France, where scientists using totally different experimental techniques reached precisely the same conclusion. Most important of all, however, was the fact that Krueger's first conclusions were published at the same time that Dr. Felix Sulman in Jerusalem was looking around for a way to get a share of research funds that had suddenly become available at the Hebrew University. It was an accident comparable to the one that first led Dr. Krueger to become interested in ions.

The Hebrew University benefits, as does so much of Israel, from the largesse of Jews in the U.S., and in 1960 the faculty received a grant from an American Jewish foundation to pay for research projects. University authorities decided that the money should be spent on projects that would contribute to a massive "Man in Israel" study. As head of a department, Felix Sulman felt that a study of the reasons why the Sharav was considered an ill wind would qualify. It did, and he and his department set out to discover why the Sharav made people mentally and physically ill and how to prevent or at least alleviate Sharav sickness.

Living in Jerusalem it is impossible not to be aware of the desert wind called the Sharav, the despair of many Israelis. As in Geneva and southern Germany, southern California, and everywhere the Witches' Winds blow, almost everything is blamed at some time on the Sharav. Murders, suicides, attempted suicides, asthma attacks, aching joints, depressions, unbearable tensions, and just "feeling under the weather" are all blamed on "the brown wind" (because it carries great quantities of sand) that blows out of the southeast for weeks at a time, and in Jerusalem sometimes for a total of 150 days a year.

Sharav is the Hebrew word for the wind known in the Arab lands as the Hamsin. The word Hamsin literally means "fifty," which indicates how many days the wind is believed to blow between spring and autumn. In most Arab countries judges are known to take a lenient view of crimes of aggression and violence committed during the Hamsin; one ancient written Turkish law actually stipulated that if the Hamsin were blowing at the time of a crime of violence or passion, it should be considered legal grounds to deal lightly with the offender. According to some translations the Old Testament, in the Book of Isaiah, refers to the Sharav as an evil, destructive, deceiving wind. The Israeli army considers the wind a natural enemy of an efficient fighting force. All officers know that if you leave men on guard duty in the desert frontier for too long they grow depressed and apathetic and suffer from a malaise the army calls "Bedouinism"—that is, they cease to be alert, effective fighting men.

The Arab races have learned to live with the Sharav, or at least to suffer it, perhaps because it is such a familiar part of their lives, just as the Foehn is to the Swiss, Austrians, and Germans. They accept it because they know no alternative. Most Israelis, however, are newcomers to the Middle East and are acutely aware that the Sharav is an unnatural phenomenon.

Felix Sulman began his work in a most unscientific manner. He told me that he and his assistants began "by listening to the gossip at the tea parties, because people were always talking about what the Sharav does to them or their husbands or wives or other relatives." Then he had the guidance of a friend, a shoe store proprietor, who showed Dr. Sulman his sales figures. "They were 300 percent higher during Sharav because people found their feet swelled and they needed a bigger pair of shoes," said Sulman. As a doctor he knew heart attacks were more common during the Sharav. Psychiatrist friends told him their patients were more troubled than at other times (which reminded me of Helen Eliat van de Velde), and an insurance assessor claimed that there was an increase of more than 100 percent in traffic accidents during Sharav. The police said the incidence of acts of aggression—wife-beating among them—and of seemingly pointless violence also went up during Sharav. Thus the research began with a list of Sharav symptoms that documented aberrant behavior and obvious physical ills.

With the basis of his earlier work in gynecology that showed the possible effects of serotonin on the human body and psyche, Dr. Sulman set out to determine the normal levels of serotonin in healthy people who were not Sharav-sensitive. He found such people on his own staff. Daily samples of their urine were analyzed to determine just how much serotonin their bodies manufactured, and how much of it was broken down by the body into a harmless substance which we'll call 5HA. (It is identified chemically by the more awesome serial number 5-HIAA.) These tests went on for four years, and the conclusion was that serotonin is not found in the urine of "normal" people except when they are under considerable emotional stress or anxiety.

Then Dr. Sulman set out to test Sharav victims. He opened a clinic in downtown Jerusalem not far from the legendary Jaffa Gate to the old walled city. Via television, radio, and newspapers he announced his study project, and asked Sharav victims to volunteer for tests. Within days he had 200 men and women, some young, some old, from every stratum of life and about every country on earth, all saying, in effect, that the Sharav made life so unbearable for them that they were prepared to offer themselves as human guinea pigs if there was any chance of a cure. For the next year the body functions of these people were monitored so intensively that they were even required to provide urine samples twice daily. Dr. Sulman found that during Sharav their body chemistry was thrown entirely out of balance, and, more significantly, that on average the victims' bodies produced 1,000 percent more serotonin during the Sharav than at other times, while their capacity to render it down to the harmless 5HA increased by only between 100 and 200 percent.

Coincidentally, Dr. Sulman had established that heat alone—during Sharav the temperature soars to 90 degrees Fahrenheit—could not produce the changes in body chemistry found during the Sharav.

What then? What was it about the Sharav that changed the body chemistry so drastically? Aware by now of Dr. Krueger's pos-ion/serotonin theory, Dr. Sulman recruited meteorologists and physicists to measure the electrical nature of the Sharav. On non-Sharav days the total ion count in Jerusalem is around normal; that is, the count is between 1,000 and 2,000 ions of both polarities. Two days before the start of a Sharav the count soars, and while the wind blows it is always at least double the normal level. And it is two days before the Sharav arrives, when the pos-ion count is highest, that most sensitive people begin complaining. Dr. Sulman told me: "Many people throughout the world claim to be human barometers. They say, 'Ah, it's going to rain because my bad knee hurts,' or 'I've got a migraine,' or just generally that 'I can feel it in my bones.' Well, I should think we've got more human barometers in Jerusalem than anywhere in the world because most of our people come from some other climate and they are very conscious of changes in the way they feel in their new homeland."

The conclusion was inescapable: The only unique characteristics of the Sharav were electrical disturbances that included massive dosage of ions, and the high proportion of pos-ions. Thus electrical phenomena in general and pos-ions in particular were the only possible explanation for the increase of serotonin production in weather-sensitive people. The bodies of such people simply cannot break the serotonin down to its harmless form.

It took ten years, but by 1971 Dr. Sulman had demonstrated that there were three distinct biochemical responses to the Sharav. The first was what he called the "serotonin irritation syndrome." Because they were, in effect, being poisoned by the serotonin produced by their own bodies, the irritation syndrome victims suffered from migraines, hot flashes, irritability, sleeplessness, pains around the heart, difficulty in breathing, a worsening of bronchial complaints, irrational tension, and anxiety. They were minor medical problems including eye inflammation and a loss of reaction time. This "serotonin irritation group" represented 43 percent of Dr. Sulman's subjects.

The second response was labeled an "exhaustion syndrome." That is, a combination of the heat and the pos-ions had, over the years, left the body incapable of responding to the stress of the Sharav. What the wind does in most people is to stimulate the body to produce adrenaline and its companion hormone noradrenaline, plus other body chemicals that generate energy and generally enable human beings to survive in the changed environment. For the first year or so this is stimulating: It produces a state of euphoria, of tingling excitement in which anything seems possible. After a few years however, the body gets tired of being incessantly called upon for an extra supply of adrenaline, and the glands lose their efficiency. Eventually, the body is incapable of producing either enough adrenaline or an adequate supply of other chemicals needed to cope with the Sharav. Biochemically speaking, its victims become exhausted. Forty-four percent of the Sharav victims were diagnosed as suffering from this "exhaustion syndrome."

And finally there was the hyperthyroid response. That is, the Sharav—and its pos-ions—throw the thyroid gland out of kilter. Since the thyroid regulates much of human behavior and feelings, the symptoms that the hyperthyroid response produces are not dissimilar to those of serotonin irritation and the exhaustion syndrome. For instance, migraine, tension, anxiety, sleeplessness, and a few other problems are common to all three types of Sharav victims. So is the overproduction of histamine, the chemical that aggravates allergies.

The fact that overdoses of serotonin are at first stimulating to many people led Dr. Sulman to argue that many tourists visiting Israel for only a few weeks found the Sharav invigorating and pleasant. He also concluded that people under thirty, whose metabolic rates are usually high and who are certainly at their fittest, react to the positive electricity by storing it like a battery until they literally become both physically and mentally overcharged. As we shall see later, in some cases this can produce an enjoyable if temporary euphoria, a belief that anything is possible. In other cases, however, it is just as likely to produce all the

problems that older, long-time residents and Sharav
victims complain about. It is worth noting here that
American researchers have found that overdoses of
pos-ions can actually make rabbits, the most timid of
all creatures, behave aggressively.

Ruth Cale, one of Israel's most seasoned newspaper correspondents, first experienced the Sharav
when she arrived in Jerusalem on April 1, 1935.
"Everybody was flopping around like dying flies," she
told me, "but I had just come and I loved it, just like
the tourists love it today, and just as some people always do. My father, for instance, he enjoys the Sharav.
But after a couple of years I began to dread it. It
makes me so foul-tempered and I feel as though I have
a cold all the time and I can't work, at least not as
much as usual. I wish I were like the wealthy ones,
able to leave town in Spring and Autumn and miss it."

Eric Marsden, the distinguished staff correspondent for the London Sunday *Times*, first moved to
Jerusalem in 1971—and instantly began to suffer from
asthma. He found that no one else was surprised. "It's
just the Hamsin," they told him. In the years that
followed he noticed that troubles between the Jews and
the Arabs along the West Bank of the Jordan often
seemed to coincide with his asthma attacks, when he
felt least able to work. "I know I'm a Hamsin, or
Sharav, victim but so is everyone else here to some
extent," he said. "People explain almost everything out
of the ordinary—fights with their wife through to
bloody riots between Arabs and Jews—by saying:
'They've got the Hamsin.' I've sometimes thought that
the really perilous time for Israel is during the Hamsin,
because the soldiers are listless and at the same time
they have hair-trigger tempers, and if the Arab armies
could overcome their own symptoms long enough to
be able to attack at the right time there'd be a bloody
shambles."

Neither Ruth Cale nor Eric Marsden, however,
suffer as much as those who volunteered to be Dr.
Sulman's guinea pigs. They are more or less typical of
the thousands who suffer without knowing why. One

of the subjects was a young woman announcer on the state radio and television network who was so badly affected by the Sharav—"I am crippled by migraine," she said—that she once fainted soon after a broadcast, and feared that she would actually do so when on the air. A woman university lecturer who had emigrated from the U.S. found that she had not only suffered from headaches, but felt "as though there was a band of iron around my chest so I couldn't get enough air" and was so tense that she felt she was unfit to drive. The wife of a veterinarian suffered from nausea and vomiting associated with migraine and had begun to take morphine to ease the pain. By the time Dr. Sulman saw her she had become a morphine addict. And the veterinarian was himself a victim of heart pains, sleeplessness, and sore eyes. Whatever their major symptoms, all these people complained of depression and anxiety during the Sharav, but believed these to be caused by the headaches, the sleeplessness, and other physical symptoms.

Defining the reason for this suffering was one thing; curing or easing it presented an entirely different set of problems. Dr. Sulman found that drugs known as MAO blockers helped people with a low adrenaline production because they slowed down the rate at which adrenaline was broken down and excreted from the body. Those people whose thyroid gland is upset by the Sharav can be helped by taking drugs that either stimulate or depress the gland's activity. But what about the serotonin victims? Since pos-ions caused the problem, would neg-ions solve it?

At this stage in his research, Dr. Sulman had been studying the problem for almost ten years. He knew that Dr. Krueger had found that pos-ion overdoses produced a higher than normal level of serotonin in the body tissues of mice, and that neg-ion overdoses "cured" this problem. Dr. Sulman mounted an elaborate series of studies to find out whether Dr. Krueger's work with small animals could be duplicated in human beings. He set up treatment rooms equipped with electrical devices known as negative

ionizers, and 300 patients were given neg-ion overdoses. Those who claimed to feel better were then
given heavy doses of pos-ions. Within an hour those
people who claimed to have received most relief from
the neg-ions began to complain of discomfort from
the pos-ions; their problems were getting worse. In this
manner Sulman reduced to 129 the number of subjects
who were clearly victims of the serotonin irritation
syndrome rather than exhaustion or thyroid malfunction. Then he embarked on another series of tests
with negative ionizers, and found that 96 of the 129
"reacted favorably"; that is, they reported that the
neg-ions eased their problems.

The fact that a few people with high Sharav serotonin levels do not respond to neg-ion treatments remains a mystery that, as I write, Dr. Sulman is still
studying. Even so, the tests proved that negative ionizers helped in almost every case where serotonin
caused people to feel physically, psychologically, and
emotionally below par. They have the same effect as
drugs designed to block the overproduction of serotonin or to help the body reduce serotonin to the harmless chemical 5HA. And those drugs, which Dr.
Sulman himself uses in some cases, often have un-
desirable side effects.

Negative ionizers—neg-ion machines—have been
in use since well before the Second World War. After
the War, however, the older designs were considered
suspect in the light of new electronic technology, and
it is only in recent years that reliable equipment has
been designed and produced. Much of the credit for
this belongs to Dr. Walter Stark, a brilliant and pioneering physical chemist who has made a modest for-
tune running his own private and profit-oriented
laboratory near Lugano, Switzerland, since he was in
his early twenties. A tall, broad man who walks with
the slight stoop common among scientists and academ-
ics, Stark has succeeded in the years since he earned
a doctorate simply by inventing things, and by being
an avant-garde scientific thinker; the sort of scientist
who lets an active imagination disciplined by logic lead

to what may seem to be a wild conclusion, then goes to work in his laboratory to find out whether the imaginative leap can be backed up by evidence. Early in my odyssey of research I found that many ion scientists were not only using equipment designed by Stark, but were also depending heavily on his laboratory findings.

Soon after the War many commercially available ionizers used a tiny radioactive isotope to generate neg-ions. These were considered dangerous (as well as being too bulky for convenient use) and were soon replaced by ionizers that produce ions through high voltage discharge. Dr. Stark perfected ionizers of this type so that now the machines most widely used in Europe and most other parts of the world are no bigger than a telephone or portable radio. Such neg-ion machines, placed on a table top, effectively ionize a living room or office; also available are larger pieces of equipment able to ionize say, a schoolroom or hospital operating theater. Dr. Stark's designs also led to the production of neg-ion generators no bigger than a paperback book for installation in cars, and trucks, and they are widely used outside North America. For reasons I'll explain later, none of these neg-ion machines are publicly available in the U.S.

Despite the importance of effective equipment, however, it is Dr. Albert Krueger, the doctor and bacteriologist, who has directed the course of ion science since 1960. His early work proved that pos-ions stimulated the production of serotonin in the bodies of small animals. That helped explain physical ills associated with distortions in the ion balance. But what of the anxieties, the depressions? Later work proved that small animals subjected to pos-ion overdoses also had an excess of serotonin in the mid-brain. And the mid-brain is known to be the control center of mood and feeling. Although he never discussed the implication in public, Dr. Krueger told me privately that ions seemed to affect the work and temperament of his assistants. Other ion scientists have used Dr. Krueger's findings to argue that serotonin overproduction caused by pos-ion poisoning is bound to affect one's frame of mind.

Dr. Krueger once departed from his usual academic prose to suggest that the ion effect is a sort of scientific bumblebee. Much of the accepted wisdom on which modern medical science depends suggests that it is unlikely that ionization could have a physiological effect, yet the ion scientist Krueger and others can observe that it obviously *does* have such an effect: Aerodynamic theory used to build all airplanes can be used to prove that the bumblebee cannot fly, yet, it does. Dr. Krueger could have made the same point by emphasizing the fact that we know that aspirin works, but we still don't know quite how or why. Doctors give it to quiet the nerves, reduce pain, and help ease fevers—but none of them knows how it does so.

In fact, Krueger himself had proved that the ion effect is not a scientific aspirin. Nor is it comparable to the flight of the bumblebee. Supported by the work of Dr. Sulman and others, he has provided widely accepted answers to those nagging "How?" and "Why?" questions that bedeviled the early ion scientists.

Many researchers suggested that neg-ions had a tranquilizing effect before Dr. Krueger actually found that pos-ion overdoses produce significant quantities of serotonin in the mid-brain of laboratory animals. The current theory is that serotonin irritates that part of the brain in people. Post-Krueger experiments have not confirmed this; in fact, such experiments on humans are at present technically impossible. But in 1965 one American scientist trained rats to press a lever in order to receive a reward of food. Once this feeding pattern was established, the scientist began to "cheat." When the buzzer sounded and rats pressed the lever, they did not always get food; sometimes they got an electric shock instead. Soon the rats refused to press the lever on cue. Instead, when the buzzer sounded they began to show all the signs of anxiety. To "cure" the anxiety and get the rats back to pressing the lever, they were fed the tranquilizing drug reserpine. The "anxiety syndrome" was depressed, and the rats merrily went on pressing levers, sometimes getting food and sometimes an electric shock. The researcher repeated the experiment using overdoses of neg-ions instead of reserpine and got precisely the same results.

In another experiment in the U.S. at about the same time rats of various ages were taught to find their way through a maze. In normal environments the younger rats learned to escape from the maze more quickly than the older rats. But when the older rats were treated to neg-ions they learned the maze as quickly as the younger ones. Not surprisingly, when given a choice, the older rats preferred a negatively ionized chamber rather than the one with normal air. The younger rats showed no preference. In rats as in humans, it seems that wisdom—or at least prudence —comes with age.

In 1969 Felix Sulman found that "normal" people—his subjects were two groups of men and women between twenty and sixty-five—became irritable and fatigued when left for an hour or so in a room that contained a heavy overdose of pos-ions. Yet the same people confined for the same period in air that contained an overdose of neg-ions showed, via the electroencephalogram, a slower, stronger pulse rate of Alpha waves of the brain than when they were in normal air. (Alpha wave rhythms are considered a measure of the brain's activity and health: A slow, firm pulse rate is generally regarded as an indication of health and tranquility and increases alertness.) He tested their alertness and work capacity by giving each of the subjects a series of alternate choice tests involving word, figure, and symbol selection. All of them scored "significantly higher" on these tests both during the time they were in a neg-ion room and immediately afterward than they did when in normal air.

At about the time Sulman was measuring Alpha waves in negatively ionized environments, doctors at the Catholic University in Argentina were administering neg-ions to patients suffering from forms of psychoneurosis that emerged as irrational apprehensions and fears. The experiment resulted in the conclusion that almost 80 percent of the patients treated "responded beneficially," frequently with a complete disappearance of symptoms. Neg-ion therapy for patients under psychiatric care but not considered clinically sick is now a standard procedure at the Catholic University hospital and at others in Argentina.

In 1971 Dr. Sulman dropped another stone in the scientific pond. He reported in several medical and scientific journals in Britain and Europe that he had experimented with several hundred human subjects and found that air ions clearly had significant biological effect on about 25 percent of the population and considerable effect on another 50 percent. The remaining 25 percent were—like Dr. Sulman himself—not troubled when the ion balance was upset. Furthermore, he had proved that, generally speaking, pos-ions are unhealthy, particularly if an individual is subjected to overdoses of them for protracted periods of time. Neg-ions, on the other hand, were generally beneficial.

By the time I met Dr. Sulman in 1972 he had almost achieved guru status among scientists who, stimulated by Dr. Krueger's original work, had been conducting experiments with ions throughout the 1960s. Sulman had even written part of a book to which Dr. Hans Selye had also contributed. In it Sulman pointed out that the Sharav was an external stress even by Selye's rigorous definitions, and that serotonin overproduction was one of the body's responses to that stress. Thus anxiety, that inexplicable affliction of modern urban dwellers, is perhaps not always due to the internal stresses of urban life and to the disaffecting pace of social change. It may be due to external stresses set up by distortions in the normal or "healthy" ionization in those environments that we have created for ourselves.

In my case, Dr. Sulman diagnosed a combination of the serotonin irritation syndrome *and* a tendency to hyperthyroidism. He gave me drugs to normalize my thyroid gland and to block the production of serotonin. He also prescribed a negative ionizer. He told me that the cases I mentioned earlier had all been cured, or at least partially alleviated. The woman radio announcer no longer feared she would faint on the air; the university professor happily drove her car and no longer complained of tension and headaches; and the woman who had become a morphine addict was cured. They were not, he pointed out, magical cures. They came about because the immigrant Israelis were more aware of Sharav problems than other people in the Middle East, and because Dr. Sulman had accepted the folk wisdom that said the Sharav was an ill wind and tried to find out why. Ultimately, with Dr. Krueger's aid, he had succeeded.

"Scientific caution is necessary, but no one can really prove in a laboratory that the bad winds really are bad because you cannot duplicate nature in a laboratory," he said. "Similarly, you cannot always rely on laboratory tests to find out what works for people, because people are not like mice or rabbits."

I left Jerusalem with my new pills and returned to Geneva and bought a negative ionizer. Within a month or so I began to feel better. I was also intensely curious. I knew I had only seen the tip of the iceberg, and I wanted to see the rest.

5

The Ion Effect
on the Human Body

As we have seen, for some Israelis, particularly those under thirty whose bodies are at their peak of efficiency, pos-ions sometimes produce a state of euphoria and optimism so strong that the people affected find it easy to believe that anything is possible. Sharav-borne pos-ions can also be stimulating to visitors to Israel. This phenomenon is not confined to Jerusalem. When I first went to live in Geneva I found the city exciting, and my problems began only after my body had been exhausted by pos-ion poisoning. Furthermore, Russian scientists are now known to believe that pos-ions are good for those people with underactive automatic nervous systems because the stimulus that produces euphoria in normal people will also bring underactive systems up to par.

This is what I have already described as the ion effect paradox. Clearly, in some cases modest overdoses of pos-ions can temporarily be good for people. And with some plants, even heavy overdoses seem to stimulate growth; they become bigger and fatter and

48

provide more food than if grown in normal ionization. But equally heavy overdoses of pos-ions seem to over-stimulate and cause harm to animals and humans.

Bishop James Pike was the controversial Episcopalian Bishop of San Francisco until he resigned in 1968, barely months before he was finally expelled from the church for heresy. He did not believe in the Virgin Birth of Christ or, it seemed, in the established church itself, and he died in the arid desert near the Dead Sea in September 1969. Felix Sulman believes he died as a result of a pos-ion overdose during the Sharav.

Bishop Pike was fifty-six when he visited Israel in 1969. He was accompanied by his third wife, thirty-year-old Dianne Kennedy, with whom he had written his most recent book. At dawn on September 3 the Israelis found Dianne staggering down the highway alongside the Dead Sea. She said her husband was in the desert awaiting rescue. She explained that "we took this ride into the desert for a few hours because we thought we might get the feel of the Judean Hills in order to explain properly the time of the historical Jesus. The car got stuck on some rocks and boulders about three o'clock. We tried for about two hours to get it freed and then we decided to leave it and walk toward the Dead Sea. We had no idea exactly where we were. My husband got tired, and I left him on top of a small mountain six or seven miles west of the Dead Sea and came on to get help." She had walked for ten hours, stumbling many times on the rocks, once nearly falling off a cliff. "It was a miraculous escape for me," she said. "I kept praying he will have the same miracle."

The Israelis and local Bedouins—all of them astonished that Pike would have embarked on a trip into the roadless desert with neither guide nor provisions and in an ordinary sedan car—mounted a massive land and air search. Five days later, James Pike's body was found only a five-minute walk from a water hole that could have saved his life. He had died of hunger, thirst, and exhaustion.

In his laboratory in Jerusalem, Dr. Sulman studied reports on Pike's behavior prior to his foolhardy trip along the unpaved pathways of the desert, and concluded: "He was a man of mercurial temperament and a febrile nervous system, the kind of person likely to be greatly affected by the Sharav. He had taken a lot of psychedelic mood-altering drugs and from his rather erratic past behavior it's reasonable to believe he already had an unstable body chemistry or nervous system. He was the sort of person who would be thrown totally out of balance by even a modest overdose of serotonin. For them to have embarked on such a trip suggests they, like most tourists, were suffering—enjoying would be a better word I suppose—the euphoria that the Sharav can bring to some people at the same time that it's causing so much distress to others. I believe Pike was more euphoric than most people ever become."

If Sulman's post-mortem diagnosis is correct, the case of Bishop Pike is a classic example of the pos-ion paradox: At first, a brief overdose can often make you feel happily hyper; that anything is possible. Even so, all the available evidence demonstrates that even if they at first make you feel euphoric, too many of them can do nothing but physical or psychological harm. However, in all the thousands of experiments conducted around the world during the past seventy years or so, no scientist or doctor has ever found that a neg-ion overdose will do anything more than keep you awake and active for longer than is normal. Ion scientists have now begun to ask *how* the body absorbs ions. Since we inhale them, part of the absorption must take place in the respiratory tracts and lungs. The details of how the body uses them and their charge are complex and not particularly well understood: As the pioneer Danish researcher Christian Bach points out, our understanding of precisely how our bodies are affected by ions is at present comparable to man's understanding of light before the prism was invented. In the mid-1960s, for instance, experiments showed that the cilia of the trachea, or windpipes, of small animals are stimulated by neg-ions and depressed by pos-ions. Human cilia, like those of small animals, are microscopic hairs that maintain a whiplike motion of about 900 beats per minute while cleaning the air we inhale of dust and pollen and other matter that should not reach the lungs. Subjected to tobacco smoke, which absorbs neg-ions, the cilia slow down. Tobacco smoke *plus* pos-ions make this slow-down take place from three to ten times more quickly than does the smoke alone. An overdose of neg-ions, however, neutralizes the effect of smoke on the cilia. Although this experiment took place in a laboratory and involved mice, rats, and rabbits, the implications are clear: Smoking and other forms of pollution that absorb neg-ions may also damage the ability of the cilia to clean the air that finally ends up in our lungs. Does that mean there is a relationship between pos-ions and the incidence of lung cancer, particularly in smokers? As Denmark's Bach points out, that is one of the many things about ionization we don't yet know, though scientists are investigating this relationship.

The effect of ions on respiration is more obvious. The U.S. experimenters Windsor and Beckett gave sixteen volunteers overdoses of pos-ions for just twenty minutes at a time and all of them developed dry throats, husky voices, headaches, and itchy or obstructed noses. Five of the volunteers were tested for total breathing capacity, and it was found that a pos-ion overdose reduced that capacity by 30 percent. Exposed to neg-ions for ten minutes, the volunteers' maximum breathing capacity was unaffected. What is significant here is that neg-ions did not affect the amount of air breathed, but pos-ions made breathing more difficult.

Ions are also absorbed into the human body through the skin. The late A. L. Tchijewsky, a Russian scientist whose pioneering ion-science work dating back to 1924 was not known in the West until a decade ago, argues convincingly that the nerve endings under the skin serve as receptors for ions and have a direct influence on the body and its organs. Dr. Walter Stark, the Swiss physical chemist and biophysicist believes that the points at which the body absorbs ions are likely to be the same as those used in acupuncture. Although this age-old medical treatment from China is now being increasingly accepted by the North American medical establishment as effective, again it is a phenomenon that no one can yet adequately explain.

It is interesting to note that Tchijewsky tried raising mice, rats, guinea pigs, and rabbits in totally deionized air. Within two weeks almost all of them died. Despite the fact that autopsies proved they had died for a variety of reasons—fatty liver, kidney failure, heart degeneration, and, among other ills, anemia— Tchijewsky concluded that the real cause of death was the animals' inability to utilize oxygen properly. He decided that vitamins and air ions had similar effects, and reported that he and his colleagues had proved that "an organism receiving the cleanest type of air for breathing is condemned to serious illness if the air does not contain at least a small quantity of air ions."

Tchijewsky's colleague D. A. Lapitsky tried raising small animals in air depleted of oxygen. As they were about to die of suffocation he added neg-ions and found that "animals already near death from asphyxiation began to feel better, sat up, sniffed the air, and began to run around the chamber. Their respiration frequency increased. Switching off the ionizer again brought them to the verge of asphyxiation." Lapitsky decided the traditional belief that oxygen alone was the sole prerequisite for the creation and sustenance of life had been "demonstrated to be false." Or as Tchijewsky said, "Death of animals in filtered [deionized] air must be attributed to the absence of aero ions of oxygen essential to the life activity of an organism." More simply put, without ions we couldn't absorb oxygen in the quantities needed to live. And the fewer ions there are, the lower the efficiency of our minds and bodies. After reviewing the scientific work of the Russians, Dr. Krueger says that they have clearly demonstrated that "work capacity, general health, and tranquility are improved by exposure to high concentrations of negative ions."

What is probably the most comprehensive and elaborate experiment ever undertaken by ion scientists was mounted in the Soviet Union, apparently soon after the end of the Second World War. A. A. Minkh, another leading Russian researcher, led a group of doctors, psychologists, and physicists in staging what might be called the Ion Olympics in which forty men and women athletes housed in special quarters equipped with laboratory facilities were put through their paces.

First, some athletes were required to lift a weight of three to five kilograms at a rate of one lift per second until they collapsed from fatigue. Having exhausted their subjects, the scientists gave them overdoses of ions. Some were given neg-ions only, some overdoses of both kinds of ion, and others were left to recover unaided. The ones given neg-ions recovered first, then the ones fed an overdose of both kinds of ions. The last on their feet were the athletes who had been left to go it alone in normal air. The same athletes were then put through the same test *after* breathing high quantities of both pos-ions and neg-ions. The conclusion was that their abilities as weight-lifters were improved by neg-ions.

Another test in the same series involved twenty-four female athletes. It lasted a month and began with a week-long series of medical, physical, and psychological examinations. The women were then split into two groups and at times were placed in sealed rooms and given overdoses of either neg-ions, pos-ions, or both kinds of ions. Sometimes nothing was added to the air at all, though the athletes were not told this.

Here it should be said that these athletes were, in fact, simultaneously undergoing a period of training and daily workouts, and an improvement in their performances would have taken place anyway. The scientists were measuring static and dynamic performance—that is, the ability to perform muscular functions while standing or sitting still, and then while in motion. The test included measuring the strength of the handgrip of the athletes; having them ride one of those infuriating machines fixed to the floor where you pedal like mad just for the joy of watching a needle move around a dial; and timing actual track and field performances as well.

Another standard test for modern athletes is their reaction time to visual stimuli. It is generally agreed that as the athlete gets fitter the reaction time becomes shorter and the response to it more controlled. The neg-ion team average reaction time shortened by 22 milliseconds, while the control group's responses shortened by only 11 milliseconds. If it seems absurd to draw conclusions from findings involving such minute fragments of time, it's worth remembering that in modern international athletic competition performances are often electrically timed to within one one-thousandth of a second. (In the 1976 world swimming championships a Canadian woman world record holder was defeated by the East German challenger by twenty-three one-hundredths of a second. In many cases there's so little difference between performances that the only way to choose a winner is by measuring factors totally invisible to the naked eye.)

The Ion Olympics continued with a dynamic performance test that consisted of running in place at the rate of 180 steps per minute until the poor subject athletes collapsed with exhaustion, lungs heaving and bodies bathed in sweat. Again there was at first little difference between the performance of the two teams, but by the month's end the neg-ion team's endurance had increased by a mind-boggling average of 240 percent. And it remained higher during the 10 days after ion treatments stopped, finally tapering off to a 38 percent increase over the team's original endurance level. The control group's endurance also improved—from between 7 to 24 percent, which was about what you'd expect after a period of training. And their endurance level returned to its preexperiment level far more quickly than was the case with the neg-ion team.

The next event was a balance test. The scientific papers reporting the Ion Olympics lack adequate description, but they do say that both teams were required to balance in precarious positions. The neg-ion team members' balance improved between 370 and 393 percent, while the improvement in the performance of the control group team increased by only 53 to 132 percent.

As part of the enterprise the scientists were required to assess individually the mental and physical state and function of the subject athletes. They reported that the effect of neg-ions on blood pressure, pulse rate, and perspiration appeared to be insignificant and had no apparent importance. However, the neg-ion team demonstrated considerable improvement in general physical and mental "tone," in cheerfulness, energy, appetite, and in their ability to sleep soundly. There also appeared to be an increase in their bodily absorption of vitamin C—a vitamin widely used, but not always with doctors' approval, as a therapy for colds, flu, and other respiratory ills.

The underlying purpose of the Ion Olympics was explained at the end of the scientific account of the experiment, where Tchijewsky concluded that "negatively ionized air in doses employed in medical practice at a number of clinical and polyclinical institutions in the U.S.S.R. can be used for increasing the physical work capacity and improving the general tone of healthy people." The postwar performances of Russian athletes in Olympic and other international competitions have astonished the world, and many have suspected that the Russians had a training weapon with which the West is unfamiliar. Are neg-ions that weapon? Perhaps. We are not sure when the Ion Olympics were staged; whether it was so soon after the Second World War that there was time to put the lessons learned into practice in time for the first postwar international athletic meetings at which the Soviet competitors were first seen to excel. Much of the Russian work remains unknown, and it was not until the mid-1960s that anyone in the western world heard of the elaborate experiments described here. And then it was only because of a book by Tchijewsky called *Air Ionization: Its Role in the National Economy,* published by the State Planning Commission of the U.S.S.R. in 1960, but not available in translation until the late 1960s.

The Ion Olympics and other tests on the ion effect have met with considerable skepticism in the scientific and medical communities. One argument of the skeptics is that while laboratory tests involving animals may demonstrate certain effects, the difficulty with trying to make judgments on the basis of human responses is that people tend to be subjective. The argument is, quite reasonably, that people in pain or discomfort may turn on a machine and want to be helped so badly that when they turn on a neg-ion generator they are led by wishful thinking to believe that they are being helped. Science knows this as the placebo effect, and it is, in a milder form, the sort of thing that may happen when some people are "cured" by faith healers. The cure is frequently only temporary and caused by the sufferer's own desire (and perhaps by a massive dose of adrenaline generated by the excitement of a "faith healing" service).

Having conceded this point, however, let me add this: People who are asleep cannot make subjective judgments, nor can they respond to external stimuli. Neither can babies under a year old be subjective; at that age they are incapable of reporting suspect findings to scientists.

In 1969 the French researcher Dr. Jouvet examined the effect of serotonin on sleep and found that overproduction (or in this case overdosage, since he injected a synthetic form of the neurohormone) often causes horrifying nightmares. It also caused his volunteers to sleep badly—that is, always on the edge of consciousness so they were not properly rested—and to wake after only a few hours of sleep. Put to sleep in a room containing a neg-ion generator the same people slept better despite the excess of serotonin in their systems.

And the babies? In 1966 at a hospital in Jerusalem, doctors performed a series of tests on thirty-eight infants between two and twelve months old. All suffered to about the same degree from respiratory problems. They were divided into two groups of nineteen, one kept as a control group in a ward without any ion change and the other where a neg-ion generator was in use.

The researchers reported that neg-ions without any other treatment—that is, no drugs—seemed to cure attacks of asthma and bronchitis more quickly than drugs, antibiotics included. They also observed that there were none of the "adverse side effects" frequently found when treating such children with drugs. They concluded that the children treated with neg-ions were less prone to "rebound" attacks" (relapses). As to objectivity, the scientific report said that the tests "demonstrated that atmospheric ions have an effect on infants, especially those suffering from asthmatic bronchitis." Less scientifically, they found that the babies didn't cry as often and as loudly when they were breathing neg-ions as they did in normal air. And there is nothing subjective about a bawling baby.

6

Ions in Medicine

I have never met Dr. E. Rehn, but by all accounts he is a brilliant surgeon and teacher, and the story he once wrote about the Red Smoke of Ettenheim and how it may have saved the lives of his patients has become a legend among surgeons in Europe. I tell it here, asking you to remember that Dr. Rehn's experiences took place in the early 1950s, *before* there was any acceptable scientific explanation for the phenomena he reported.

For many years Rehn had been a leading surgeon in Freiburg, near Munich in southern Germany, where he also taught at the university medical school. Like many of his colleagues he was burdened by the fact that in the Foehn-plagued area of southern Germany the old saying "The operation was a success but the patient died" is too often true. Statistically, in and around Munich there are more postoperative deaths caused by thrombosis and other blood problems than elsewhere in Europe. Either heavy transfusions are needed, or the patient's exhausted body mysteriously produces clots of blood that travel through the arteries to clog either heart or lungs. There are, of course, many circumstances in which there is both heavy bleeding and thrombosis, both potentially fatal.

In 1952 Rehn was appointed head of neurosurgery at Ettenheim, about twenty-five miles from Freiburg. He later wrote that after several years he "noticed much to my amazement that there were hardly any cases of thrombosis." He went on to say that it seemed an incredible state of affairs since there were so many cases just a few kilometers away at Freiburg. What was it? The climate? The food? The mineral content of the water? Rehn shrugged off the mystery and went on operating, happy in the knowledge that at Ettenheim his patients stood a better chance of survival than at Freiburg.

One of the minor irritants suffered by hospital staff and the people of Ettenheim was pollution from a nearby processing plant. Its smokestacks belched great clouds of red-tinted smoke that often lay like a pall over the town and surrounding countryside. It was a singularly insidious form of pollution, since after being washed and hung out to dry a few times all light-colored fabrics would take on a gentle red tint, and this alone enraged local people to the point where their demands to clean up the plant forced the company to install smoke filters.

In the town, housewives and the others who had protested against the pollution were delighted. But at the hospital, postoperative patients began to die in greater numbers. For the first time Rehn noticed that he was beginning to lose about as many patients from postoperative thrombosis at Ettenheim as he had at Freiburg. No statistics were kept and a precise cause and effect was impossible to establish. There was only one scientifically significant fact to weigh when seeking an explanation: Prior to the factory clean-up a Dr. W. Spitzer had taken measurements of the air electricity in Ettenheim and had found that at the time the red smoke was at its worst there was "a very large negative electrical charge" in the air.

In and around Munich doctors have for decades canceled all but the most vital emergency surgery

when forecasters predict a Foehn condition, that is, a
wind that would bring a heavy pos-ion charge. It is
part of local medical wisdom that during the Foehn the
patient is more likely to die, either on the operating
table or soon afterward.

If the pos-ions of the Foehn are bad for surgical
cases, then the neg-ions of Ettenheim—probably
caused by smoke coming from furnaces burning material with a high level of radioactivity—seem to have
been good for them. But why? What is it that makes
pos-ions so harmful in these circumstances, and neg-
ions apparently beneficial?

It may be possible to find at least a clue to the
answer in the seemingly unrelated findings of two
American surgeons. First, Dr. Norman Shealy, a neu-
rosurgeon and head of the Pain Clinic at La Crosse,
Wisconsin, reported early in 1976 that he had conducted a survey among fellow surgeons and found that
severe bleeding in surgical patients is widespread during periods of the full moon. He was quoted by a
newspaper as having said: "I have checked with blood
banks all over the country and I have been told that
the demand for blood transfusions is always highest at
the time of the full moon and the two days following.
Surgeons should definitely not perform any surgery except emergencies during the full moon." The second
surgeon is Dr. Edson Andrews, of Tallahassee, Florida. He is reported as having kept careful records of
1,000 patients that he operated on, and to have found
that 82 percent of all excessive bleeding took place
around the time of the full moon.

Neither surgeon is suggesting anything mystical;
nor is there any astrological implication. What is involved is one of the mechanisms that affects the ionization of the air.

The major source of ions in the air within a few
hundred feet of the surface of the earth is the radioactivity of the ground and the rays of the sun. However, there is a little-understood interplay between the
earth itself and the ionosphere, the layer of charged air
and particles that envelops the earth about seventy-five

miles up. The ionosphere absorbs much of the sun's harmful radiation and thus makes life as we know it possible. This protective belt is not only charged electrically but also polarized, so the underside that faces earth is positively charged and the top, which faces outer space, is negative. The interaction between the positively charged underside of the ionosphere and the negatively charged earth is probably a key element in the generation of ions of both polarities and in the maintenance of the balance between pos-ions and neg-ions.

The moon orbits the earth outside the ionosphere. Like the earth, it is negatively charged. When the moon is full it is closer to the earth than at any other time and repels the negative outer face of the ionosphere. Thus the ionosphere is pushed closer to the earth, and the interaction between the positively charged underside and the negatively charged earth means that when the moon is full, or nearly full, the number of pos-ions close to the earth's surface increases.

Again, we don't need to look far into the accumulated wisdom of humankind to know that the lunar cycle affects human behavior. It is enshrined in the word "lunatic," and countless scientific studies conducted throughout the world demonstrate that aberrant human behavior is most common at the time of the full moon. Those people already sufficiently mentally disturbed to have been committed to mental institutions are more restless at the time of the full moon than at any other. And we now know that pos-ions cause an overproduction of serotonin; that serotonin is a stress neurohormone; and that among the more weather sensitive of us it can upset our mental and physical equilibrium. The precise nature of our response depends on the particulars of our individual physiology and psychology. While most of us may simply be troubled, some even become explosively and irrationally violent. A University of Miami research team led by psychiatrist Arnold L. Lieber analyzed 2,000 murders committed in Dade County, Florida, between 1956 and 1970 and announced that the high peaks of the homicide rate coincided with phases of the full and new moon.

This "lunar connection" gives some clue to the vast potential medical uses of the ion effect. Recent work of scientists both in America and Europe suggests that pos-ions are a contributory cause of blood problems, and that neg-ions (remember the high negative charge of the Red Smoke of Ettenheim) cancel out the often fatal pos-ion effect. The early "natural philosophers" recognized that pos-ions had an influence on the human body, on animals, and on plants. Not knowing of the existence of ions, they suggested that "positive air electricity" stimulated the mysterious lymph fluid that circulates through the human lymphatic glands and ducts—a circulatory system that many medical scientists believe to have existed in animal life forms before they evolved to the point where blood and a vein-and-artery circulatory system came into being. Precisely how important the lymphatic system is to animal life remains a mystery, although it is known that many kinds of cancer spread from one part of the body to another through the lymph glands, and that these glands and ducts are part of the total circulatory system that carries body chemicals to the place where they are needed.

The natural philosophers also argued that at the time of the full moon there is a greater than usual positive charge in the air and that at such times the metabolic processes of life are accelerated. Seeds, for instance, germinate more readily at such times, a fact long enshrined in traditional agricultural practice and now explained by Dr. Krueger and, among others, by the U.S. agronomist who grew cucumbers almost twice as long as usual in an atmosphere with a high pos-ion content. For centuries, surgeons have felt that it was unwise to perform surgery on hemophiliacs at the time of the full moon.

Within the past decade scientists have suggested that our red blood cells absorb the air we breathe while the white cells pick up the electrical charge of that air. White cells control the blood clotting mechanism of the body, and are normally negatively charged. Because they're all charged the same way, they repel one another and don't readily coagulate or clot unless the body requires them to, as it does to help heal an open wound or incision. An overdose of pos-ions—like that in the air around Munich at the time of the Foehn—could mean that white blood cells lose some of their normal negative charge; the repelling effect diminishes and they are more likely to cling together to form clots that could cause post-operative thrombosis. On the other hand pos-ions stimulate the metabolism and that alone could be responsible for an increased flow of blood from an open surgical wound. Whether the problem is thrombosis or hemorrhage depends on the patient. In any event, at certain times and in certain places, the pos-ion overdose may throw the entire circulatory system out of balance.

This is a necessary simplification of a complex biophysical process and no scientist I know would proffer it as the definitive explanation of postoperative complications and deaths. Yet both laboratory experiments and the practical experience of surgeons suggest that pos-ion overdoses have a "bad" effect on the blood of patients after surgery, while neg-ions are generally beneficial.

Russia and the nations of eastern Europe seem to be ahead of the rest of the world, with the possible exception of Switzerland, in researching the effects of ions on blood circulation. In Hungary, operating theaters and postoperative recovery wards are commonly equipped with neg-ion generators as a matter of course, and in Russia their use in hospitals is widespread. In the West, however, medical scientists have only recently begun to test the standard practices of eastern European surgeons.

In some Swiss hospitals neg-ion generators are also installed in delivery rooms and postdelivery recovery rooms. Doctors there believe that at the time of delivery most of the mother's body is drained of its healthy bioelectric potential, all the energy being focused on the area of the womb. Again, thrombosis is one of the most common threats to the life of a woman giving birth and in the hours immediately afterward. Neg-ion generators are used because in tests they appear to lower the number of deaths during childbirth, and also appear to help the exhausted woman regain her strength, energy, and mental well-being afterward. Again, the moon appears to play a role. One of Canada's most experienced surgeons told me, "If there is a full moon due early in the two-week period when birth is expected, you can take bets on the baby being born early rather than late. I know from the phases of the moon when the busy time of my month will be." This same doctor believes that the moon may also be involved in the body chemistry changes that bring on labor pains. "One of the great mysteries of obstetrics is what actually causes the baby to be born—what mechanism in the body induces labor and so on," he says. Many obstetricians and midwives echo this man's experience, and commonly point to the fact that the time cycle of female menstruation roughly approximates that of the moon.

All this, however, comes under the unscientific heading of "empirical conclusions"—that is, while experience may show a phenomenon to be generally true, it is scientifically discounted until the questions *why* and *how* are answered. It is a characteristic of modern science that while doctors practicing the art of healing use their empirical conclusions, scientists tend to pooh-pooh the older "folk wisdoms." Yet there is much to be learned from such traditional knowledge. For example, modern antibiotic wonder drugs are really a form of mold, and one of the oldest known treatments for an open wound is to pack it with moss and other mold-creating herbs.

Until recently the situation was, of course, much the same with the ion effect, although even before Dr. Krueger's serotonin findings were published in 1960 some compelling empirical evidence of how ions can be used in medical treatment came from Philadelphia. There the work on burn victims at the Northeastern General Hospital by the late Dr. Igho Kornblueh was carefully documented with the aid of other doctors, surgeons, and electronics experts and, since it was so clinically and scientifically respectable, the results had a major impact on the world of medicine.

During a six-month period between 1958 and 1959 the hospital staff mounted a study of the effects of negatively ionized air on 187 patients—96 women and 91 men—suffering from burns of varying degrees of severity. Forty-nine of them made up a control group and were treated with traditional painkillers and other drugs. The remaining 138 underwent neg-ion treatment.

Of the 138, only 59 appeared to be unaffected by the neg-ions at the end of the six-month period. The remaining 79 were all observed to have benefited both in the easing of pain and discomfort, and in healing. That is, the conditions of 57.3 percent of the neg-ion patients improved by all medical definitions, while the conditions of only 22.5 percent of the drug-treated control group improved by the same degree in the same time. Statistically, the odds are 1,000-to-1 that this could have happened by coincidence. Even so, the doctors and statisticians were cautious in presenting their findings. They said they had demonstrated that neg-ions are an *aid* in the treatment of burn patients; that they lessen discomfort and exert a tranquilizing effect. The report concluded: "The probability that such data could have occurred by chance is remote. In view of these findings, it appears that a significant number of patients can be made comfortable even during that critical period after surgery without the use of sedatives or narcotics."

When the report was made public at the conference of the International Society of Bioclimatology at the Royal Society of Medicine in London, the Northeastern Hospital's chief surgeon, Dr. J. B. Minehart, who had been largely responsible for putting into practice the neg-ion therapy devised by Dr. Kornblueh, said, "At first I thought it was voodoo. Now I'm convinced that it's real, and revolutionary." In later years Kornblueh, Minehart, and their colleagues conducted other experiments that produced more dramatic proof of the way neg-ions eased or eliminated pain, but that 1958–59 experiment, which ended twelve months before the publication of Dr. Krueger's serotonin findings, was so convincing that the hospital's postoperative wards were promptly equipped with neg-ion generators.

Even so, there is still controversy whether the neg-ions did their work because they were inhaled or because they were absorbed by the skin and damaged tissues, or both. At first, some doctors argued that the tranquilizing effect was the most significant, since a tranquil patient is likely to feel less pain and to heal more quickly, and that the ions were only absorbed by means of respiration, not through the tissues of the skin. Others argued that only the pain-killing effect came from the tranquilizing property of the inhaled ions, while the healing of the wound itself was speeded up by neg-ions absorbed through the tissues. Supporters of this latter argument pointed out that in severe burn cases there was none of the putrid smell usually associated with such injuries.

Once Krueger's serotonin findings were published, other theories were advanced. One was the notion that the stress caused by the burn itself triggers the overproduction of serotonin, and that this excess of serotonin in the damaged tissues causes great pain. Neg-ions, so this theory goes, either suppress the production of serotonin, or at least enable the body to break it down to the harmless form I have earlier called 5HA, thus easing the pain. The same arguments would apply, of course, to all surgical cases.

Whatever the precise mechanism of the neg-ions and their effect on the burn victims, the results were unquestionable and many more experiments were conducted. By the late 1960s Dr. Kornblueh was able to be far less cautious in his wording: "Between 1956 and 1966 over 200 patients with various kinds and degrees of burns received negative ion therapy in the surgical department of the Northeastern Hospital. It was applied in all cases independently of other appropriate systematic measures as needed in individual cases. The out-patients received five times a week one treatment of twenty-five to thirty minutes duration. Hospital patients were exposed two or three times daily for a total of one to one-and-a-half hours. With rare exceptions, no analgesics [pain killers] were needed. In the great majority of these cases a complete cessation of pain was achieved after the first ten to fifteen minutes." He went on to state categorically that the healing was much quicker, that the scar was much "tidier" and that there were substantially fewer infections of the burns than is usual.

In the fall of 1971 I visited Dr. Kornblueh at his home in a suburb of Philadelphia, and found a tall, slender, gray-haired and very gracious man. He was then in his late sixties or early seventies, and was a disheartened and angry man. I had done sufficient research to know that Kornblueh was widely regarded as one of the postwar pioneers of ion therapy, though he had no satisfactory explanation of how the ion effect worked until the time of Dr. Krueger's serotonin findings. By the time we met, Dr. Kornblueh had completed what he considered his life's work—a demonstration that neg-ions had a beneficial effect on people with burns, on postoperative conditions, and on respiratory diseases. Quite reasonably, he believed that the results of his experiments would prompt other hospitals and surgeons and doctors to follow his lead. They did not do so, and it was this that caused his anger. "What more do they want?" he asked me. "God, the results speak for themselves, and the reputations of the doctors and surgeons and hospitals involved mean there just can't be any quackery. Healthy caution I can understand because, after all, medicine as a profession has a massive responsibility. But this . . . this blindness is just as dangerous to the public as a lack of caution would be. It means that a treatment we have shown to work over and over again is being denied people who are sick or injured and need it."

Igho Kornblueh died soon after we met, and today his work is quoted more often than when he lived.

Slightly less scientific but rather more interesting evidence supporting the neg-ion burn therapy came from England. Claire Maxwell Hudson, a television show host of distinctly visual charms, spilled boiling water down her stomach while making tea one morning, receiving second-degree burns. This catastrophe was duly reported in the gossip columns of newspapers, but a few months later she was able to reassure her public. She said that she owned a neg-ion generator (which she had bought to treat a mild case of asthma); that she had held it up against the burn itself three times a day; and that after a couple of days the pain disappeared and the burn began to heal. Within two weeks there was no scar to be seen. "I was absolutely thrilled," she said. "I thought I'd never be able to wear a bikini again."

One side effect of Dr. Kornblueh's experiments with burn victims was that those patients who also had respiratory problems—chronic bronchitis, for instance, or asthma—all reported that neg-ion therapy helped them breathe more easily. As a result Kornblueh mounted another series of experiments, this time involving respiratory ills, at the Northeastern Hospital, at the University of Pennyslvania's Graduate Hospital, and at the Frankford Hospital in Philadelphia, as well. He was able to report that 63 percent of patients suffering from hay fever or bronchial asthma "have experienced partial or total relief" because of neg-ion therapy. One hospital doctor who worked on Kornblueh's project said later, "They come in sneezing, eyes watering, nose itching, worn out from lack of sleep, so miserable they can hardly walk. Fifteen minutes in front of the negative-ion machine and they feel so much better they don't even want to leave." It was this, along with the other results, that led Dr. Kornblueh to coin the now widely used phrase "vitamins of the air" to describe ions.

We saw in the last chapter that the U.S. experimenters Windsor and Beckett proved that pos-ions make breathing more difficult. This experiment, and others like it, demonstrate the validity of the accumulated human wisdom that says people with respiratory problems should be sent to sanitoriums and spas known from experience to be good for such illnesses as asthma, pneumonia, silicosis, emphysema, and tuberculosis. Ion counts in such places show a high incidence of neg-ions that comes from the sun shining through high, clear air, from waterfalls or radioactive materials in the ground, or simply because in hilly and mountainous areas the air is usually cleaner and contains smaller quantities of the airborne particles that should not reach the lungs.

In the past quarter-century the spas and sanitoriums of the world have stood almost empty, partly because drugs have been found to cure or ease tuberculosis and other respiratory ills. At Davos, Switzerland, for instance, the once-famous and bustling spa hotels stand forlornly deserted and sometimes shuttered. Lately Davos and similar resorts have begun to enjoy a revival in popularity among those who suffer from asthma and hay fever and other respiratory ills usually caused by allergies that cannot be treated with drugs. The high neg-ion count in spa climates helps people breathe more easily.

The Russians often use drugs and ion therapy together, frequently sending sufferers to sanitoriums in hilly areas. Ion science pioneer A. L. Tchijewsky measured the ion levels at many Russian spas and found that all had more neg-ions than pos-ions. He suggested that this was in part because the air was cleaner and the neg-ions, which diminish when there are a lot of particles in the air, survive far longer.

The Department of Health, Education and Welfare says there are 10 million emphysema victims in the U.S. More than one million people diagnosed as incapable of working because of pulmonary emphysema are drawing social security benefits that total a staggering $60 million each month. This apart, the Department says that between 3 and 5 percent of total population—that is, between 6 and 10 million people —suffer from bronchial asthma so badly that it causes total or partial disability, and the cost in lost productivity and social support payments of one kind or another hasn't yet been computed. None of these figures includes those with chronic bronchitis and respiratory allergies, though government officials concerned with the subject operate with an estimate that more than 20 million Americans suffer from chronic respiratory problems of one kind or another. What is perhaps most significant is that these figures are rising annually. Illnesses once considered occupational hazards for miners and other workers exposed to dust have now become a national problem for huge numbers of people, regardless of occupation.

For all the clear evidence that air ions are useful for treating those with breathing problems, it is in fact often easier and cheaper to use an ionized, or charged, water spray as a medical treatment. This is known as aerosol therapy, and in North America was pioneered by Dr. A. P. Wehner, who set up his first clinic in Dallas in 1961, where he treated approximately 1,000 patients before moving the clinic to the state of Washington. He has the sufferers lie in reclining garden chairs in a closed room, and then turns on a machine that produces a massive spray of tiny droplets of water that have been electrically "charged." In almost all cases he uses a negative charge. For thirty minutes the patient lies there breathing these vaporized water "ions." This is done twice a day for a twenty- to thirty-day period. Wehner, widely recognized as a knowledgeable medical scientist, reports that he has treated people with bronchial asthma, the various types of bronchitis, pulmonary emphysema, laryngitis, pharyngitis, dry hacking cough, infections of the upper respiratory tracts, and nasal and sinus conditions caused by allergies. Based on the first 1,000 cases in Dallas, he has reported that symptoms completely disappeared in 30.3 percent of the cases; there was a significant improvement in 42.3 percent and some improvement in 20 percent. Only 7.4 percent of the patients failed to benefit in any way.

Wehner argues that aerosol therapy is more efficient than ion therapy in cases where people require medical treatment, since the tiny droplets are more easily breathed in and are more likely to get as far as the lungs themselves, carrying their electrical charge with them.

For all this, Wehner's treatments have been surrounded with controversy, a fact reflected in one of two scholarly papers he published in the *American Journal of Physical Medicine* in 1969. He wrote, "New modalities and techniques are often controversial, and this is especially true in medicine where the critical attitude of most physicians inhibits the proliferation of dubious therapeutic methods. The application of air ions and electro aerosols in clinical medicine seems to have met with particular skepticism, even though the international literature abounds with reports claiming various physiological effects of these agents. In part, this skepticism may date back to the exploitation of patients by charlatans selling worthless electrical gadgets as panaceas; in part it may have been caused by poorly documented claims, particularly in the older literature; by inconsistent results and by the fact that some of the reported findings could not be reproduced by other investigators." Dr. Wehner then proceeded to cite the newer scientific work as an argument why this skeptical attitude should now be abandoned, and ion and aerosol therapy adopted for a wide range of ills that beset mankind, respiratory ailments among them.

There is always a lag between any discovery and its practical application. It is only fair to point out that the caution of the medical profession has on occasion saved the public from danger. It was this ingrained conservatism of the medical authorities that spared the U.S. the horrors of the Thalidomide disaster that blighted the lives of thousands throughout Western Europe and Canada.

When I met Dr. Wehner he was, like Kornblueh, a disappointed man, though he had great faith that the weight of evidence supporting ion and aerosol therapy was growing to the point where it would soon spill over from the scientific literature into the public consciousness, and that once this happened the world of medicine would be forced to take a more active interest. Like Kornblueh and Krueger—indeed, like most of the men and women I've met involved in ion science—I found Wehner given to reason rather than rhetoric. I suspect, though, that at times all ion scientists are forced to take heart from the fact that people once laughed at Columbus, condemned Darwin, and called Louis Pasteur a crank.

Wehner's results are typical of many findings by European, South American, South African, and Japanese doctors. In Britain two Oxford University statisticians conducted a study among 100 victims of asthma, bronchitis, and hay fever chosen at random from a list of people who had purchased neg-ion generators in the hope that they would help their problems. In the end their report was based on interviews with only 74 of the 100. They found that 18 of 24 asthmatics; 13 of 17 bronchitis sufferers; 11 of 12 hay fever victims; and 6 of 10 people afflicted with nasal catarrh reported that the neg-ion generators had noticeably improved their condition. A few claimed the generators had cured them.

There is evidence to suggest that, where neg-ion generators are readily available, the public is far less skeptical than scientists and some doctors. In Meissen in East Germany a factory doctor set up a neg-ion therapy unit for workers whose jobs exposed them to the possibility of developing a serious lung disease. After a few weeks the workers were so impressed by the feeling of overall well-being induced by the after-work sessions that they began to ask if their wives and children could come, too. Within seven months the clinic had outgrown its original purpose. Doctors in the city began sending patients suffering from bronchial asthma and other such ills for treatment at the factory. Some even sent children with whooping cough, elderly people with emphysema, and even men and women suffering from eczema, a skin disease. Neg-ions helped all of them, presumably in the same way it helped Philadelphia's burn victims. Within two years other industrial plants, particularly smelting companies and mining operations, had begun to set up their own neg-ion clinics for workers.

By 1975 one East German doctor, who had by then treated more than 11,000 people with neg-ion therapy, said that his patients reported "with monotonous regularity" that the therapy worked. Brazilian hospitals have commonly used ionizing devices for the treatment of breathing problems, including allergies, following a test involving 36 children with asthmatic allergies. All of them had consistent and in some cases crippling problems before taking neg-ion therapy; during the treatment only one of them suffered an allergy attack and afterward all were reportedly cured, at least to the point that they no longer suffered problems so long as they took part in occasional neg-ion therapy sessions.

In my own quest for people who suffer as I did from pos-ion poisoning I came across Mrs. Patricia McDonald, a high school teacher who lives in Tunbridge Wells, south of London. She told me that she began to suffer from a form of hay fever and dust allergy after the birth of the first of her three children in 1966. Soon it had grown so serious that she could not do her own housework because the dust made her sneeze incessantly, made breathing difficult, and gave her blinding headaches. She also gave up baking at home because flour dust produced the same symptoms. "It was," she said with the understatement typical of the British, "quite inconvenient. I mean, in order to keep the place clean we had to hire help and I had to sit in the garden while the dusting was being done. Besides, I was rather proud of my pies and cakes and the family liked them, too." Perhaps to save on the housekeeping bills, or to ensure his supply of pies, Mrs. McDonald's husband, Richard, an electronics

engineer, acquired a neg-ion generator. It worked, at
least to the degree that Mrs. McDonald is now back
doing her own dusting and baking. When last we
spoke she said, "When we got the ionizer in 1970 I
would sit down beside it and the help was almost immediate. It was almost as though someone had touched
me with a magic wand. I'm one of those people who
responds to it quickly, and now I seem to be more or
less cured. But it's still useful. I put it in the children's
rooms when any of them is ill, and it helps a lot with
croup [dry cough] and those awful English colds that
produce so much horrid mucus. They sleep better, too,
which makes life easier for me."

In 1970 Dr. Harry L. Beckman of Bedford, New
York, applied Dr. Kornblueh's lessons to another medical problem that also had significant economic implications—bedsores. He was treating patients in the spinal
cord injury unit of a hospital in Westchester, where
the injured spend weeks, even months, lying prone
as part of their recovery treatment. He found that the
resultant bedsores often lengthened his patients' stay in
the hospital, taking up needed beds and, with ward
care costing several hundred dollars per patient per
day, draining the hospital coffers. In his scientific findings he pointed out that there is no known cure for
bedsore ulcers, and that they are apparently a problem in all hospitals and convalescent institutions. But
Dr. Beckman decided to try something he called
"oxygen ion therapy," in which a plastic bag placed
over the bedsore was filled with oxygen heavily
charged with both pos-ions and neg-ions. Dr. Beckman concluded that "preliminary clinical impressions
give every indication that oxygen ion therapy has
proved to be successful in all patients."

The limited promotion that ionization has received as a medical treatment has too often tended to
be mere proselytizing by those who, having "discovered" it for themselves, have been overly enthusiastic, often leaving the impression that they're promoting
the ion effect as a magical cureall. One example is
the fact that many migraine sufferers, who make up

somewhere between 7 and 10 percent of the population, have somehow come to believe that neg-ion generators are the cure for their own particularly durable and treatment-resistant headaches. They are not. They do, however, help in many cases, and as I write the Migraine Trust of Great Britain is midway through an elaborate series of experiments involving two major British teaching hospitals to determine just how neg-ion generators can best be used in treating this affliction.

These experiments are inspired by the experience of Dr. Peter Fox, of Dorchester, England. A man in his late fifties, Dr. Fox is both a general practitioner and the superintendent of a children's hospital, and is himself a victim of what he describes as "a particularly vicious form of migraine." By 1971 his attacks—between thirty and forty of them a year—had grown so severe that from the onset of a migraine headache he would suspend medical practice and "make sure I had someone with me at all times because, frankly, the pain was so severe that I felt I was not responsible for my actions and might well jump out the window or run for the nearest shotgun." After reading medical journal reports of Felix Sulman's work in Jerusalem, he bought a neg-ion generator and was so impressed with the way it eased his problem that he promptly acquired two more, one for his office and one battery-operated model to use in his car, and when on vacation. In the three years since, he says he has had only one migraine attack, and that was instantly eased by retiring to a room where the ionizer was turned on.

As he tells it, "Migraine is not a modern problem since it was mentioned in wall writings in the Tomb of Thebes built in 1500 B.C., but I'm under the impression that the number of victims has increased rather a lot in the past twenty-five years, or at least since I've been practicing. On the other hand, because I'm a sufferer myself perhaps people with migraine tend to seek me out as a doctor because I'm more likely to be sympathetic; it is, after all, a problem very difficult to understand if you've never experienced it. In any event, when I found this machine worked for me I began trying it out on migraine patients. During the three years since I first heard of Sulman's work I've concentrated where possible on treating migraine victims, and I'm fairly sure now that I can diagnose the commonest migraine of all, Acute Migrannus Neuralgia, or Horton's Migraine. It's the one form of migraine —there are seven or eight that we know of—that turns up in men as often as it does in women; women, you know, make up 70 percent of migraine cases. Well, once I was fairly sure I could diagnose Horton's Migraine I started suggesting patients with it get themselves an ionizer. I treated fifteen or sixteen patients and scored thirteen direct hits, though there was one case when I was sure the ionizer would work and it had no effect at all."

When in the fall of 1975, Dr. Fox reported his findings to the Migraine Trust, they decided that the neg-ion treatment was worth a full-scale scientific examination. Six months later one of the researchers told me cautiously that the early results were "quite encouraging."

I have found that victims of the Foehn often complain of migraine headaches along with other ailments, and Dr. Sulman reports similar findings. On the face of it, the connection between serotonin and migraine seems obvious: A stress neurohormone that is found in the mid-brain and is known to cause anxiety and a host of other problems related to the psyche is quite likely to be the cause of the severe and crippling headaches that are clinically diagnosed as migraines.

Of all the research now underway into the nature of the ion effect, the most potentially dramatic is in the area of cancer. We have seen how experiments demonstrate that a healthy dose of neg-ions is vital to keep the cilia of the respiratory tract working at maximum efficiency, thus quite possibly helping to prevent lung cancer. But this is only one area of research relating to cancer. Clarence D. Cone, a N.A.S.A. researcher, has found that the surfaces of cells of the body carry a negative charge. In healthy people that charge is more or less the same in all cells, and Cone suggests that normal cell development and interaction is only possible while the charge remains the same. The rogue cells of a cancerous growth, however, have a far lower "negative potential"—that is, capacity—than healthy cells. By some mechanism we cannot yet begin to understand, those rogue, low negative-energy cells can multiply—and kill. Cone's discoveries suggest that it may be possible to increase the negative energy potential of cancerous cells and, in restoring them to normal, "cure" cancer.

Since the cells apparently get a large part of their electrical charge from the ions we breathe and perhaps absorb through the skin, it was inevitable that scientists in the U.S. National Cancer Institute now reportedly investigating Cone's discoveries should consider the ion effect. Many cancer researchers, having worked for years on chemotherapy and immunology as possible cancer cures, now consider the work inspired by Cone as the most promising new area of investigation.

Cone's discoveries will be of paticular interest to the Russians, who apparently have been trying for years to find a link between cancer and air electricity. Most of their experiments, as reported by Tchijewsky, have been inconclusive, though one experiment involving mice had intriguing results. Following an established laboratory technique, a group of mice were injected with cancerous cells. Six of them were removed from the group and placed in an insulated cage—that is, the cage was not grounded to earth. Thus they were suspended in the air electricity with no way for the energy to be conducted to earth. All six mice developed what is known as spontaneous regression of the cancer. Within six weeks five of them lost the cancerous swellings completely and lived for several months longer than any of the other infected mice. No one draws any conclusions from this experiment, beyond the obvious one that air electricity appears to be involved in the development of cancer in mammals.

Ion therapy has become an important and widely used tool in Russian health services. Having earlier mentioned "therapeutic doses" of ions used in medical practice, Tchijewsky reported that ion therapy using both total ion overdoses and overdoses of neg-ions in particular was only of "particular benefit" to people with pulmonary tuberculosis, bronchial asthma, hypertension, joint disease, sinusitis, migraine, and diseases of what he called the "peripheral nervous system." This is the same as the vegetative nervous system mentioned earlier—that part of the nervous system programmed by genetic history to control all the unconscious bodily functions that keep us alive: heartbeat, respiration, kidney function, liver, blood pressure, digestion, and among other things, the production of body chemicals like serotonin as we need them. Many researchers in the U.S. and Britain as well as in Russia have suggested that one medical problem caused by either ion starvation or an unhealthy imbalance between pos-ions and neg-ions is "neuro-vegetative dystony"—a catchall phrase used by doctors who, while they can't say why, know you have an illness caused by a failure or malfunction of this vegetative nervous system. Such illnesses may be explained by Dr. Krueger's discoveries that pos-ions produce serotonin. We can, however, be sure that ions have a significant influence on the hypothalamus, the master gland that produces many of the body's control mechanism chemicals and has a direct effect on the brain, the bones, the blood, the spine, the liver, and on the gonads in men and the ovaries, menstrual cycle, and lactation in women.

It seems likely that changes in serotonin production caused by variations in ionization hit first at the weakest part of an individual's body—the "target organ" in medical language. Thus a man with an old war wound will first feel the effect of an upset ion balance in the area of that wound; someone with a weak liver will suffer worsening of the condition that already exists; a woman who has given birth by Caesarean section will probably feel discomfort in the region of her womb and perhaps her genitalia. Almost everybody reading this will have some medical problem, however minor, that is periodically rather more bothersome than usual. That sudden flare-up of an old ache or a sore back or a so-called trick knee may well be due to an otherwise unnoticeable change in the pos-ion to neg-ion balance, and perhaps—in certain cities and climatic conditions—a sudden increase or drop in the total ion count. The sudden worsening in the condition of patients of my analyst friend Helen Eliat van de Velde is, as I said earlier, probably explained by a change in the weather.

Despite the skepticism and debate over the value of ions as a medical treatment, there is one ion effect that has, in parts of Europe at least, quietly crept into public acceptance—the ionizer as an air cleaner. Dust and pollution particles attract neg-ions and, to a lesser extent, pos-ions as well, which then transfer their charge to the particles. These charged particles form clusters and are too heavy to remain suspended in the air and fall to the ground as dust, or are drawn to the walls of any room or building.

Using ionizers to clean the air in this way is, in a sense, a crude adaptation of Dr. Krueger's first discovery in the field of ion science—that is, that neg-ions have a biological effect on bacteria and, in killing these germs, clean the air. Again, there is some disagreement about the precise mechanism. Since the time of Krueger's major breakthrough in this field, many researchers have shown that actual bacterial growth in laboratory petri dishes is slowed and even halted by neg-ions. It is, however, also suggested that bacteria, staphylococci, and other airborne germs that spread common respiratory diseases attract ions so that they, too, form clusters and fall to the ground, just as dust does. Whatever the actual mechanism, the effect is clear. One post-Krueger experiment shows that the "decay rate" of bacteria in natural air is only 23 percent per minute, while in air treated with pos-ions the rate is 54 percent. In air treated with neg-ions, however, the decay rate goes up to 78 percent per minute. In 1963 Russian experimenters claimed that concentrations of around 10,000 ions of both charges per cubic centimeter completely exterminate the most common disease-carrying bacteria. This seems to explain why one result of the neg-ion therapy practiced on the burn victims in Philadelphia is a reduction in the incidence of wound infection.

For almost as long as I can remember, North America has suffered from a plague of one form of contagious influenza or another just about every two years. It spreads throughout the big cities, and the infectious germs are carried around the country in cars, trains, buses, and planes. As I write, an epidemic of a particularly vicious form of influenza called swine flu is being predicted. If we lived in environments that had a normal balance of pos-ions and neg-ions, we might be spared some of the agonies that are sure to come. But the man-made twentieth-century Witches' Winds mean that most of us spend most of our lives in ion-depleted air, one of the obvious consequences of which is that infectious germs live longer, thus allowing diseases to spread more rapidly.

7

Our Man-Made
Ion Prisons

One sunny day in the summer of 1972 I called at the gleaming new office building housing the Rothschild Bank in Paris and was told that the department I wanted had decided to move back to the old and comfortably decrepit building from which the bank had moved months earlier. When I finally caught up with the man I sought, I asked what was so wrong with the splendid new offices. "None of us could stand working there," he said. "Everyone started getting colds and felt badly all the time, and since our job isn't part of the front office business we moved back." He went on to list the complaints that his colleagues had made about the new building: feeling off-color and tense, lacking energy, and being depressed and headachy. He said the complaints stopped when they moved back to the old, drafty, brick office block they'd worked in for years.

Could a building cause symptoms similar to those spawned by the Foehn, the Sharav, and the Santa Ana? Could air-conditioning systems be creating twentieth-century Witches' Winds? A year of research later, using the knowledge of thermodynamics I had obtained in my training as a mechanical engineer, I knew not only that I was right, but that the man-made environments of the Age of Technology are a potential threat to everybody, not only to those who, like me, are weather sensitive. Sprawling cities, automobiles, pollution, smoking, modern synthetic fibers from which our clothes and furnishings are made, new building materials, modern transportation, and above all the central heating and cooling systems in hermetically sealed high-rise office and apartment buildings—all of these are part of man-made environments that have too few ions of both kinds for healthy, normal life.

In humid areas—New York in high summer, for instance, or in Toronto—part of the familiar discomfort is caused by the fact that air becomes ion-depleated. Really humid days are murder for anyone suffering from asthma or any respiratory allergy, and the fact that such people find it difficult to breathe in hot, humid air may have less to do with the amount of oxygen in that air than with massive neg-ion depletion. Air electricity is quickly conducted to the ground by the moisture in the air, and what neg-ions there are attach themselves to particles of moisture and dust and lose their charge. We have seen how pos-ions make breathing difficult and reduce the body's ability to absorb oxygen; and how neg-ions help breathing and improve oxygen absorption.

The ion count is always low in cities where there's precious little open ground to generate them. Pollution makes a bad situation worse, since it tends to deplete the neg-ion count even more. The high pollen count in certain parts of North America each fall cuts even further into the neg-ion count, since pollen has the same effect as dust. The end result is that the total ion count in cities is always down to what many scientists consider perilously low levels. As if that weren't bad enough, the normal 5–4 ratio of pos-ions to neg-ions is distorted so that people are, in a sense, eternal victims of pos-ion poisoning.

Certainly the 60 percent of North Americans who live and work in cities and urban areas are suffering to a greater or lesser extent without realizing why, although they are often conscious that *something* is amiss. But if, like the staff of the Paris bank, they work or live in centrally air-conditioned and heated buildings, their feelings of apprehension may reach quite frightening proportions.

Hot or cool air forced through duct work of most central heating and air-conditioning systems sets up friction that results in the loss of almost all the neg-ions and also draws most of the pos-ions out of the air as well. Then comes the coup-de-grace: This air with some pos-ions and virtually no neg-ions is forced out through vents into rooms, offices and passages—and as it passes through the vents more friction is set up that generates an additional overload of pos-ions. What finally comes out of most heating or air-conditioning outlets in the offices we work in and the rooms we live in is likely to be an eternal Witches' Wind likely to upset the mental and physical equilibrium of everyone, not only those of us who are ion sensitive.

Just how bad these systems are depends to a great extent on their design and the materials from which the duct work is made. The design or layout of the whole system is crucial. At bends and curves and right-angle junctions the friction between ducts and air increases and has the effect of increasing the number of pos-ions in the air. What comes out of the heating and cooling vents in any centrally heated or air-conditioned building is air that is not only low in total ions, but also has a heavy pos-ion count when measured against the almost negligible quantity of neg-ions. It is because of the design of this duct work that some parts of a building may be more "uncomfortable" to work in than others. This depends on whether you're on the receiving end of air that has passed through a particular section of duct work, where there is a sharp bend near the outlet—as the air is forced around bends and corners there is greater friction and a consequent increase in pos-ions. I have a friend who was so uncomfortable in one high-rise office that he moved —to the room immediately next door. There he felt, as he put it, "more or less human again." I suspect there was a bend in the duct work between the two rooms. The problem may be as bad in a suburban split-level or a single-story office building, but it is obviously likely to be even worse if you work or live high up in a skyscraper. The air has farther to travel to the fiftieth floor than to the second. The only way you can tell whether your office or home is particularly unhealthy is by finding someone with the know-how and equipment to pay a house call with an ion-counter.

Simply by occupying a room we can make a bad situation worse, since in confined spaces for prolonged periods of time people consume ions faster than they are created in the "dead" air of sealed buildings. Breathing and smoking do it—and so does just moving around. Most modern offices and apartments are broadloomed with synthetic fiber carpeting that, as we set up friction by walking across it, tends to generate a positive charge in the air. And then most of our furniture and drapes and clothes are of synthetic fabrics of one kind or another, and these worsen the situation. Only a fabric made from cotton creates neither a positive nor a negative potential, while the most commonly used synthetics create a positive potential— that is, when worn or walked on the friction involved generates a positive charge and positive ions. Try pulling a shirt or dress of synthetic fabric over your head on a dry day. With no air moisture to conduct the positive charge generated by the friction to earth, that charge causes the garment to cling to your body. But more of that later; for the moment let us consider the consequences to human health and happiness.

Early in 1975 I met a journalist from the *Ottawa Journal,* a newspaper in Canada's capital where a large slice of the nation's civil servants work in a forest of relatively new office buildings that are usually both air conditioned and centrally heated. The reporter and I talked of the ion effect, and as a result she asked whether she could use our conversation as the basis for an article. A few days later, the *Journal* carried a front-page story that mentioned very briefly some of my findings about the way we distort the ion balance in modern buildings. To everyone's astonishment, the newspaper received a flood of confirming letters and phone calls from civil servants.

Some readers even called me in Toronto, almost 250 miles from Ottawa, seeking more information. This reader response prompted the newspaper to run a second front-page story, which read in part: "Employees at the Department of National Health and Welfare are literally gasping for air. So much so that many leave work early feeling headachy and dizzy or 'stuffed up.' Apparently the situation is no better at the House of Commons. Or in at least a dozen steel and glass air-conditioned offices where windows are permanently sealed. The *Journal* was besieged with telephone callers Friday following a Thursday report that ion-depleted air caused by air conditioning may be the source of a multitude of ailments cropping up in Ottawa's work-a-day world."

Reporter Karen Moser went on to quote government social worker and consultant Ted Blake as saying that the air in the 16-story building in which he worked was insufferable. He apparently said: "Around two p.m. the air smells like a closet which hasn't been aired for weeks. I get headaches and dizzy sometimes." And this is just a sample of a dozen or more interviews reported by the newspaper. In all, the response to the original story was so unprecedented that the *Journal* arranged for Rosemary Dudley, head of the Toronto-based Migraine Foundation, to take the calls. They even went to the trouble to publish a front-page notice to announce that fact. Dudley knows enough about the ion effect to field questions and make suggestions about how the problems might at least be eased.

Nine months later a friend in London told me of a similar situation there. In England neither air conditioning nor central heating is quite so vital to survival as it is in North America, and so it is only recently that London (and the rest of Europe for that matter) has been blessed with these hermetically sealed high-rise archetectural horrors that are so common in the U.S. and Canada. One of the most recent and impressive groups of such buildings is the complex built by the giant International Publishing Company on the south bank of the Thames in London. One of the editors of a major women's magazine owned by the IPC told me that within weeks of the company's move to the new complex from old buildings scattered around the city, unrest among the staff, due to the "climate" in the new buildings, had grown to such proportions that both management and unions became involved. The staff complained of precisely the same things as the group in Paris, and the Ottawa civil servants: headaches, colds, inability to concentrate, and depression. The management was as puzzled as anyone else by such complaints from sane, intelligent people at the top of a tough profession. Had they been aware of the ion effect, they might have responded to some obvious clues. One editor found her office more habitable when she sprayed the air with water, and for no apparent reason and in all weather, nearby decorative fountains became a favorite place to gather at noon and eat a sandwich lunch.

It is a measure of the general ignorance of the ion effect that no one—not the unions or the management—considered the possibility that the people asked to work in this great air-conditioned beehive complex were suffering from ion starvation, and possibly from pos-ion poisoning. For instance, within weeks of the move there was an increase in sickness among the editors, writers, photographers, clerks, and typists who populate the skyscrapers for a third of their daily lives. Why this should have happened was—and perhaps still is—a mystery to management, unions, architects, and staff. Yet elsewhere many earlier experiments have demonstrated that heating and cooling systems in sealed buildings cause problems with worker morale and health.

Most of this research has been done in Europe, though some experiments have been conducted in the

U.S. One of them involved offices of a Swiss bank branch office in New York. The actual test was conducted from January to March of 1973, at a time when there was an epidemic of what was dubbed London Flu. Neg-ion generators were placed in two working areas, both of which had sixteen people in them, and were left running throughout the three-month period. Members of the staff were told they were "air cleaners"; there was no mention of neg-ions and their virtues. At the end of the test period it was found that of the thirty-two employees, only nine were absent for two or more days and that a total of fifty-three days' work was lost through sickness. The year earlier during the same three months and at a time of a similar epidemic (this one called the Hong Kong Flu), every one of the thirty-two people on the staff was off for two days or more at some point, and a total of eighty-nine days of work was lost. The statistics in themselves may be faulty—perhaps one kind of flu was more virulent than the other—but the bank management sounded impressed when they reported the results to the Swiss manufacturers of the ionizing equipment.

It is the man-made Witches' Winds, not the ion effect itself, that is of crucial importance in the continuing history of humanity. Mankind evolved in air that is rarely "ideally" ionized. That "healthy" ion level of 1,000 to 2,000 ions per cubic centimeter with a 5–4 ratio of pos-ions to neg-ions is found over an open country field on a clear day. But even in nature total ion count and balance fluctuate, sometimes wildly. There are more ions in the woods than in fields; more on a sunny than a cloudy day; more where the ground has a high radioactive content. The weather, the moon, and the seasons all affect both the ion count and the balance. The human system, like all living things, can and has coped effectively with these occasional fluctuations and regional variations in natural ionization. When the ion count would go down to an unhealthy level or the balance was distorted, our ancestors were not permanently affected because neither circumstance would last long. Where level or balance was permanently unhealthy because of, say, radioactive materials in the earth or rocks, they could learn from experience that it was an unhealthy area and would usually avoid settling there. Yet today an estimated 60 percent of the population of North America spends about 80 percent of its time in cities and urban areas where the total ion count and balance is hopelessly and perhaps permanently depleted and destroyed.

As many scientists have pointed out, humankind evolved over the great maw of time in "normal" ionization, and consequently we are all bioelectric creatures designed by nature to function properly in an environment that contains a certain level of air electricity. Humans can, and have, adapted to myriad changes in their environment, and have to some extent been adapting to artificial environments ever since they learned to use fire. Yet not until the past century were they required to adapt to a totally man-made environment, and not until a quarter century ago did heavily and constantly polluted urban sprawl and hermetically sealed centrally heated and cooled buildings come to constitute the environment in which most men and women (at least in the West) spend most of their lives.

The works of Hippocrates, father of modern medicine, contain many references to climate and air and its effect on human well-being. He said that "south wind induces dullness of hearing, dimness of vision, heaviness of head and languor." Almost all the Witches' Winds found in nature are from the south. The man-made Witches' Winds don't blow from the south; they may also blow from wherever the air or heating vent happens to be located. In medieval England, a house not located so that it was not exposed in some way or another to winds and breezes that would renew the air (and thus the ions) was considered to be a "bad" house. In 1671 the English natural philosopher Bohun wrote that architects should consider giving freer admission to the winds "since it has been observed that several dwellings here in England which were environed with huge woods or sometimes had only a clump of trees set towards such a quarter [the direction from which the prevailing wind blew] have always been obnoxious to sickness till they happen to be cut down; then the place is rendered pervious to the winds. Sometimes only the changing of a window or door from the south and exposing it to the north has done a great cure. It is well observed that in relation of my Lord Howard's Voyage to Constantinople that at Vienna they have frequent winds which, if they cease long in summer, the plague often ensues, so it has now grown into a proverb that if Austria be not windy, it is subject to contagion." (Vienna is also plagued by a Foehn condition, and is said to be part of a "Suicide Belt" that stretches up through middle Europe where, when Witches' Winds blow, the suicide rate soars.)

If all this were true *before* the age of smoking factory chimneys and great industrial sprawl that covers up land with buildings and asphalt, how much more true is it likely to be of today's cities? Over open country, air contains around 6,000 particles—pollen perhaps, or dust—per milliliter of air. In the industrial cities of North America and Europe the particle count soars to *several million* particles per milliliter. And particles—dust—eat ions; or, rather, they destroy the small ions that have a physiological effect, and tend to destroy more neg-ions than pos-ions. Measurements reported by scientists show that at main intersections in Leningrad, Paris, Zurich, Munich, Dublin, and Sydney, among other places, the small ion count is usually reduced to an average of between 50 and 200 at midday. Scientists in Zurich and in Munich took an ion count in the downtown areas at noon one sunny day and found only 20 ions per cubic centimeter.

Back in the mid-1950s when entrepreneur-manufacturer Wesley Hicks first persuaded Alfred Krueger to take up ion science, he also commissioned electrical engineer John Beckett to measure ionization. In one test Beckett set up a bank of measuring equipment 350 yards from the Bay Bridge approach road in San Francisco. He left the equipment running for 24 hours, and when he checked its recorded ion counts, decided at first that the machines were faulty. Years afterward he told me: "There was a funny fluctuation in the morning and early evening. At first I suspected the equipment, but when it checked out O.K. I repeated the tests and found that during the morning and evening rush hour traffic on the freeway the small ion count totally disappeared. There simply weren't any to be counted."

In the mid-1960s Krueger mounted a complex ion science experiment with the support of the Pollution Control Office of the Department of Health, Education and Welfare, one of several federal agencies that at times helped fund his work. This particular experiment involved keeping the inevitable mice (Krueger steadfastly refuses to conduct any experiments involving humans) in various ion levels and balances of air. For his experiments he defined ion-depleted air as an environment containing between seventy and eighty pos-ions and eighty to ninety neg-ions, and he found that in such air the mice caught influenza more easily and died from it more often than in "normal" air. In a published report, Krueger, ever the cautious scientist, permitted himself a modest speculation. "So far as environmental factors are concerned," he wrote, "man encounters for long periods of time certain of the air ion concentrations we imposed upon our mice. Should he live in the congested area of a typical city, toil in a factory where gaseous and particulate pollutants are generated freely, or work in an ordinary office, it is certain that the air surrounding him will be ion depleted. People traveling to and from work in polluted air, spending eight hours under the conditions described above and living their leisure hours in urban dwellings providing essentially the same ionic microenvironment [as that in which the mice lived] inescapably breathe ion-depleted air for a very substantial portion of their lives." Krueger has not suggested what the consequences might be, except to say that "Living in ion depleted air is clearly unnatural, and therefore presumably unhealthy."

What that evidence clearly suggests is that the

human capacity to adapt to environmental changes may be immeasurable—but we clearly could not adapt to life without oxygen or vitamins. And ions—healthy ion totals and balances—clearly have an effect analogous to both.

The effect of ion depletion in a closed space was first demonstrated empirically in Japan in the late 1930s. While much of the detailed conclusions drawn from experiments conducted at that time are questionable in the light of modern technology, the Japanese work is still frequently quoted by ion scientists, perhaps because of its magnitude. Researchers in the faculty of medicine at the Imperial University at Hokkaido began experimenting with people in an ordinary room, but by 1938 had escalated until they were working with a movie house holding an audience of 1,000.

A room was specially prepared so that temperature, humidity, and oxygen content could be controlled, but the ions could be slowly removed. Then fourteen men and women ranging in age from eighteen to forty were introduced to the room and spent some time getting comfortable in it. While temperature, humidity, and oxygen level were all kept at optimum "comfortable" levels, the ions were removed. The subjects began to complain of a variety of problems from simple headaches through dizziness and excessive perspiration to feelings of anxiety. In some cases they were even found to have lower blood pressure than normal. All said the room felt "stuffy"; that the air was "dead."

Another group of human subjects were sent to the movies, where in a crowded theater the effect of smoke and great masses of people sitting close together means that the small ion count grows very low. When the movie ended the moviegoers all reported that they felt much as we all do when leaving a theater—a mild, but not particularly troublesome headache, and slight perspiration. They were promptly put in a room where a neg-ion generator was at work, and all reported that within minutes they felt better;

their headaches were gone and the perspiration ended.

Next the Japanese scientists decided to wire the entire theater for ions. First, they sent their sample people into a crowded movie house. When half of them began to complain of the mild headache and perspiration common among moviegoers, the scientists started pouring neg-ions into the auditorium from several locations in the roof and walls. They held the neg-ion count at between 500 and 2,500 per cubic centimeter, and after 90 minutes of the movie those who had reported headache and perspiration said that both symptoms had disappeared and that they felt about the same at the end of the film as they did when it had begun.

I have perhaps done the scientists involved a disservice by condensing their findings. In fact, the tests took place over a period of eight years and were far more complex than I have suggested here. The conclusion was that brief exposure to air ion imbalances and depletion had little effect on people in normal health, but that even an hour or so in such environments could exert a "remarkable" effect on those with subnormal health or disorders of the nervous system. Like so many others before and since, these researchers reported that "positive ions had a tendency to produce stimulating effects, for example, sleeplessness, headaches, discomfort, an increase in blood pressure and pulse rate . . ." On the other hand, neg-ions in reasonably low concentrations "exerted sedative effects, namely sleepiness, soothing and quietness, calming the itch, checking the sweat and the decrease of blood pressure, producing a decrease of pulse rate, a decrease of blood sugar . . ."

But how long does a movie last? Even Stanley Kubrick's epics end in four hours, and we emerge to a more or less normal environment. That's not the case if you work in an air-conditioned or heated office, or live in such an apartment, or—heaven help you!—do both.

In January 1975, the British Society of Environmental Engineers were told by C.A. Laws, an electrical engineer, and Dr. E. R. Holiday, a medical doctor, of the effects of pos-ion overdoses on animals and humans in natural environments—the Foehn, the Sharav, and so on—and in laboratories. They said that similar and frequently worse environmental situations were created by prevailing conditions in cities and industrial areas, and in centrally air-conditioned and centrally heated buildings. "Indoors, the situation is made worse by the action of air ducts in trapping further ions, principally negative ones, and by the effects of people breathing in a confined space," said the engineer and the doctor in a jointly written scientific paper. "Smoking provides a further source of condensation nuclei. The net effect is that large numbers of city workers spend their days breathing air with typically just 200 to 300 positive ions and 150 negative ions per cubic centimeter as compared with between 1,000 and 2,000 of each sign in clean country air."

They went on to say that people affected by city environments—particularly people like me who are weather sensitive—might be expected to experience similar symptoms to the Sharav-sensitive patients of Sulman in Jerusalem; that is, tension, depression, reduced work efficiency, and headache or "heaviness," these conditions worsening as the day progresses. To a greater or lesser extent, nearly everyone will be similarly affected. The tension and weariness after a "hard day at the office" that drive you to have an after-work drink or lead to a fight at home may have less to do with your job and the workload then the artificial climate in which you have spent the previous seven or eight hours.

It must be said here that Mr. Laws, a man with a distinguished record as a pioneer in radar systems and in the automation of British heavy industry, is in the business of manufacturing neg-ion generators and Dr. Holiday is a consultant to his company. However, I have spent a considerable amount of time with Laws, and found him the antithesis of the proselytizing salesman or entrepreneur. A small, balding man who smiles so rarely that it seems like a benediction when he does,

"Coppy" Laws is, if anything, the classic image of the back-room scientist come to life. Along with Dr. Holiday he spent the first part of the 1970s trying to encourage other scientists to do new work that would produce yet more evidence to prove the critical importance of the ion effect. Even so, Laws is sometimes more sought after than seeking: Ionizers designed by him have been requested by many hospitals and industrial concerns that have grown aware of the ion effect through word-of-mouth promotion. Early in 1976 I investigated two cases where his ionizers had been in use for a year or longer. One was in the control room of the Essex County police headquarters, and the other was at a plant producing precision measuring equipment.

The police control room is in a century-old red brick building in the ancient town of Chelmsford in eastern England. The control room is fourteen feet by eleven feet and it is manned at all times by eleven men and women, who operate the communications and radio equipment. For years, the officers who staff the control room worked there happily, but technology conspired against them so that by 1970 their working conditions had become, as Superintendent Malcolm Moore told me, "bloody impossible." The radio equipment grew more complex and a computer terminal was installed—both pieces of equipment that, like Wesley Hicks's original electric heaters, generate massive overdoses of pos-ions. Then the room was broadloomed with synthetic fabric. The officers wore uniforms tailored from partly synthetic fabrics, and all were issued with nylon shirts, so they were wearing clothing that both generates and picks up a heavy positive static charge. Supt. Moore told me that whatever they tried—fans, air conditioners, dehumidifiers, and so on—the room was always heavy with smoke, smelled of perspiration "and had something about it so that at around two o'clock in the morning it was just about impossible for anyone to stay awake, let alone alert and on the ball. Everyone was complaining of headaches and a sort of draining tension. The drowsiness was noticeable and quite unnatural; I even worked the night shift myself to find out what the staff was talking about." In the spring of 1974 a neg-ion generator specially designed by Laws for large offices and rooms was installed. Now Moore says that the problems have all disappeared and "things have improved so much now that we get people complaining they can't get their forty winks in the middle of the night because they don't feel like it."

The problem at the industrial plant was both similar and yet greatly different. There, in the town of Crowborough in southern England, the Taylor-Servomex plant produces delicately engineered oxygen sensors in what, in industry, is called a "clean room" —that is, a working area where the air is washed, filtered, cooled, cleaned, and so doctored that it is as pure and particle free as air can ever be. In this case between twelve and fifteen people worked at any one time in the "clean room," and management reported that they were unhappy doing so. Riad Kocache, the head of research for the company, explained that "the air goes through a heating cycle and pipes and filters and we were getting only positive ionization." One worker complaint was that this impeccable air was "stuffy"—an echo of the complaints of the Japanese subjects who, spending time in a room with perfect air, complained of discomfort.

At around the time new machinery was installed in the room the Taylor-Servomex company also hired Laws to install a neg-ion generator in the air purification system. When we spoke, research director Kocache was cautious in his conclusions. Yes, he said, the neg-ion generator did seem to cancel out the excess of positive ions; in fact, the ion ratio was now one of slightly more neg-ions than pos-ions. Yes, some of the operators did seem to think that their working conditions were better, though others could see no difference. Yes, it was true that some of the workers said they actually felt better since the neg-ion generator was installed. And yes, production did go up, although that might be due to the new manufacturing equipment. No ecstatic endorsements of neg-ion generators from Mr. Kocache. But as our conversation ended he said, almost reluctantly, "It seems to have helped keep people happier and certainly seems to have helped them work more efficiently." It was as though Kocache, a scientist, was reluctant to concede the value of neg-ions before their beneficial effect had become an accepted scientific wisdom.

Similar caution—indeed, skepticism might be a better word—was displayed by Barry Blain, a researcher working for the British government's Police Scientific Development Branch who was given the job of finding out whether neg-ion generators might be of benefit in all police installations—as they were at the control room at Chelmsford, Essex—and in other areas where personal comfort and alertness are vital to crime prevention and control. In his final report he referred to only 5 of the 5,000 or so scientific papers and articles that I know to have been written on the ion effect. After reporting that "it is clear there is little agreement among the specialist workers in the field on the exact biological effects of airborne light ions," he noted that "there is evidence that under certain circumstances an appreciable reaction occurs in complex systems, such as man" to changes in both ion count and ion balance. And he did concede that at least one probable effect of using neg-ion generators in man-made environments was a reduction in airborne pollution from dust and cigarette smoke, since ions convey their charge to such particles and are either drawn to the walls, floor, or ceiling of the room. He also conceded that ionizers appeared to reduce the build-up of static electricity in a building, with a consequent reduction in "the unpleasant electrical effects"; and that they caused a reduction in the number of bacteria carrying infectious diseases. On the latter point he wrote: "It is possible that the toxicity of negative ions to certain microorganisms could cause a reduction in the susceptibility of subjects to some ailments."

However much they beg the question, even congenital Doubting Thomas scientists are now being forced to reluctantly concede the point that neg-ions are good for you and pos-ions are, generally speaking, unhealthy. Here it is probably necessary to stress again that in most people not actually suffering from a respiratory or nervous problem, the most noticeable beneficial ion effect is to repair the damage done by man himself to the air we breathe and the world we live and work in. In many, perhaps most, offices, factories, and homes neg-ion generators are generally necessary to return air electricity to something approaching normal, at least in terms of the ratio between pos-ions and neg-ions. Clearly, except in certain medical conditions mentioned previously, neg-ions are unlikely actually to cure anyone of anything. Their most noticeable effect, however, is to give us more energy, both mental and physical, and improve our mental and physical well-being.

I am myself astonished at the skepticism of people like Riad Kocache and Barry Blain. The weight of evidence on my desk about the visible benefits of the artificial generation of neg-ions in modern urban environments is overwhelming. Leaving aside for a moment all disagreement about just what ions actually do to living organisms, consider these random items:

In 1932 Dr. C. W. Hansell, a research fellow at the R.C.A. Laboratories in Camden, New Jersey, noticed a startling swing in the behavior of a fellow R.C.A. scientist who worked beside an electrostatic generator. Some days this man finished work full of energy, vitality, and in irrepressible good spirits. On other days he ended his day by being rude to colleagues and friends, ill-tempered, and depressed. Such swings in mood and manner were alien to the man and his nature, and the change seemed to coincide with his move to that particular location in the laboratory. Out of concern for his friend, Hansell investigated, and found the scientist was happy when the electrostatic generator was adjusted to produce neg-ions and morose when it was producing pos-ions. As a result of this accidental discovery, Hansell went on to become a distinguished ion scientist.

In one major Swiss bank the staff was divided

into two groups, one of 309 men and women and one of 362. The first group worked in offices where the air was treated to turn the normal ion balance on its ear— there were, in fact, more neg-ions than pos-ions. The second, and larger group, worked in untreated air. The test period lasted for several months, and at the end of it the ratio of days lost due to respiratory illnesses— colds, flu, laryngitis, and so on—by both groups was measured. The conclusion was staggering. For every one day lost among the group of people working in neg-ion enriched air, there were sixteen lost among the people working in normal air.

In a world-famous Swiss textile mill a smaller study produced even more startling statistical findings —and in such cases as this it is worth noting that the workers were not asked for their subjective responses; all the results were based on days lost through work. In this instance for six months in the winter of 1971– 72 ionizers were installed in two rooms, both sixty feet by sixty feet, in each of which twenty-two people worked. During that period one neg-ion generator was switched on but the other was permanently turned off. In this manner both groups were led to believe they were working in an environment where the air had been enriched with neg-ions. That winter a total of twenty-two days was lost through sickness among those who worked in the room where the ionizer was working. But sixty-four days were lost among those who worked in the room where the equipment was never turned on. During a month-long flu epidemic the neg-ion group lost three working days; the other group lost forty. The statistical conclusion was that, since the only change in personnel and working environment was the generation of neg-ions in one room, the ionizers alone were responsible for a 92.5 percent reduction in time lost through common winter maladies.

The basement of the Standard Bank of South Africa in Johannesburg houses the data processing room. Ninety-one operators, almost all women, work the electric calculators and computers necessary for such an enterprise. They process checks and vouchers worth $200 million each day. Staff unrest at the working conditions grew so bad that the bank, almost in desperation, installed neg-ion generators, not really convinced at the time that they were likely to help matters. Two years later a management spokesman said that the ionizers were obviously good for the environment, and that the operators' error rate had dropped from 2.5 percent to 0.5 percent. "You can't *see* the effect, except that in a sense you can," he was reported as saying. "You can see it in the improved standard of work and the improved feeling of the workers."

Another South African bank copied the Standard Bank's example in its computer room and reported similar results. There a supervisor said that they had even added piped music to the data processing room to keep the staff there happy, but that still they had complaints of headaches and found that the employees were grumpy and irritable and apparently took it out on their families and friends when they finished work for the day. Until the neg-ion equipment was installed, that is. Then the absentee rate went down; the staff turnover slowed from remarkably high to more or less normal, and general morale was reportedly "high—everyone even seems happy."

The case histories seem endless. When a neg-ion generator was installed at a kindergarten in suburban London, the incidence of colds and sniffles went down and the children appeared to be more "aware" and able to learn more easily. At least one captain commanding a U.S. nuclear sub won't put to sea unless he has neg-ion generators in his cabin and on the "bridge." Soviet scientists told to devise the best possible artificial environment for space capsules found that any enclosed compartment with "conditioned" air is likely to be low in total ion count, that such ions as did exist were most likely to be pos-ions and that a prolonged stay in such environments is "likely to be detrimental."

Scientific measurements? In 1972 Dr. S. Tycza told the International Symposium on air ion therapy in

Budapest that he had just completed a study of measurements of air ionization in 650 "working and living spaces" in his native Poland. One segment of his report dealt with the ion count in three kinds of offices—one that was unheated and ventilated simply by opening a window, one that was heated but still ventilated by opening the window, and one that was in the kind of tightly sealed building that has proliferated in North America in the past quarter century. In each case the offices were of a similar size and each was occupied by five people. In the unheated office with the window, there was at the end of a working day 92 percent of the outdoor ionization. In the heated office that had a window which could be opened, the ionization at the day's end was 74 percent of that outside. In the office that was hermetically sealed and heated, the ionization had dropped to just 51 percent of the ion count outside. (Dr. Tycza's report to the Budapest symposium dealt with total ionization, not with the distorted ion balance in the buildings studied. It seems likely, however, that had he measured the ion balance he would have found—as did Dr. Walter Stark and I when we made random measurements in New York in the summer of 1972—that there were almost no neg-ions present at all. Dr. Stark and I took a portable ion counter into a half-dozen centrally air-conditioned skyscrapers in Manhattan and found only pos-ions.)

Should the Polish study be suspect because the work was done in an eastern bloc country, let us consider the findings of the research department of the U.S. Federal Aviation Administration, the Washington –based agency responsible for air traffic safety. By 1970 the F.A.A. had received many complaints from air traffic controllers that when working at radar consoles they suffered irritating sensations around the face, nose, and eyes. Since most plane crashes take place when aircraft are either approaching or leaving airports, and since the controllers are the people who direct these parts of the flight by using radar equipment, the problem was considered sufficiently serious to put a team of scientists at work at the F.A.A.'s experimental center in Atlantic City, New Jersey.

In 1972 they produced a report two-and-a-half inches thick. In it, much of the scientific work done by Krueger, Kornblueh, Sulman, and others was examined and reviewed. The conclusion was that modern radar equipment may produce a new and hitherto undetected ion that is smaller than usual and has its principal effect on the exposed skin of the face. This ion would not have the same biological effects as other ions since it would not survive as an ion long enough to be inhaled far into the trachea and lungs. The researchers did not state that this ion constituted any danger to air traffic safety, although they did report that "it would appear desirable to maintain an awareness of the ionization conditions of the atmosphere in the controllers' working environment." However, their other findings were of major significance.

For instance, the F.A.A. scientists wrote at one point: "The atmosphere is our most precious natural resource. Since we all breathe air from the day we are born until the day we die, and since atmospheric ions have been shown to exert significant effects on living organisms, the fact that there is relatively little ongoing research concerning their physical nature and behavioral, physiological, and biochemical effects seems appalling." They later added: "Atmospheric ions can affect the health, well-being, efficiency, emotions, and mental attitude of human beings. The particular effect varies with the polarity and size of the ions. Negative ions are being called 'happy ions' whereas positive ions are being called 'grouchy ions.' "

As we shall see, the F.A.A. scientists also had something to say about the importance of a healthy ion balance in aircraft cabins and cockpits, but their summation of the importance of the ion effect to human physical and mental well-being is succinct and specific. You don't have to be one of the 25 percent of the population who are weather sensitive to be bedeviled by man-made Witches' Winds. To a greater or lesser extent, as we have seen, every one of us is influenced. If we were subjected to an overdose of pos-ions for a period of just a few days, or if we were required to spend just a small part of our lives in an ion-depleted atmosphere, the problem would not be so great. But, I repeat, the accepted statistic is that 60 percent of us live in cities and urban areas where the ion count is already lowered by pollution, and we spend not a few days or weeks but 80 percent of our lives in such places. No one knows what proportion of that 60 percent of the population who are city dwellers also works or lives, or does both, in hermetically sealed, air-conditioned, and centrally heated buildings. But it is high; higher in the U.S. and Canada than anywhere else in the world. These people are working and living in an unnatural environment deprived of anything resembling "normal" air electricity—one of the major factors in the evolutionary process that, through the millennia, created us in the image we are now.

The social scientists—psychiatrists and psychologists mostly—have for a decade now been talking about the epidemic proportions of a condition they describe as "anxiety." They have argued that anxiety is part of the human condition and that a degree of it is healthy, even essential to human survival. That is, you should be a little anxious about keeping your job because that way you'll try harder and be more successful; you should be a little anxious about the happiness of your wife or husband or current love because if you are you'll go to greater lengths to please them. Psychologist Dr. Martin Seligman of the University of Pennsylvania points out that anxiety is a component of human growth and progress, and may even have first emerged in evolutionary history when early man sought shelter in caves by night, when the beasts of a primordial world ruled the earth.

However, social scientists now show an alarming degree of unanimity in their belief that the base level of anxiety within the human race has gone above the "healthy" level; that we are all, for one reason or another, subject to so much anxiety that it takes very little—just a fight between husband and wife; an abrasive encounter with a cabbie or a neighbor; a thoughtless word from a colleague or the boss—to overload the system and cause a fuse to blow somewhere in the psyche.

An anxiolytic is a drug designed to ease anxiety —the oldest known of which is alcohol. The statistics about the increase in the consumption of liquor, wine, and beer and the consequent increases in alcoholism have been quoted so often it would be superfluous to repeat them here. But along with booze, we have become chronic pill poppers, and most of those pills are tranquilizers designed to ease or decrease anxiety. In 1974 almost three billion Valium and one billion Librium tablets, the most common tranquilizers, were consumed in the U.S. alone.

And yet all the symptoms described by people who can be proved to be victims of pos-ion poisoning are the same, or similar, to those that people report when they go to see doctors, psychiatrists, and psychologists and complain of what may be medically described as anxiety psychoneurosis. Think of the symptoms that I experienced in Geneva; that Sulman's Sharav-victim patients reported—insomnia, irrational anxiety, inexplicable depression, constant colds, irritability, sudden panics, fits of absurd indecision, uncertainty. At the Catholic University in Argentina one doctor took patients he considered classic anxiety cases and treated them with neg-ions in a closed room. All had earlier complained of the unnamed fears and tensions typical of anxiety psychoneurosis victims. After between ten and twenty sessions, each lasting fifteen minutes in the neg-ion therapy room, 80 percent of his patients reported that their symptoms not only disappeared during treatment but also did not recur between sessions.

Consider the facts: In cities and urban areas there is ion starvation; in air-conditioned and centrally heated buildings there is both ion-starvation and pos-ion poisoning; and almost all the cases of anxiety psychoneurosis now being dealt with by doctors are in cities and urban areas. Neither I nor any ion scientist would suggest that the obvious conclusion is necessarily the correct one. There are many possible reasons for the fact that anxiety has become perhaps the major problem besetting North Americans. But the new awareness of the ion effect should cause psychiatrists and others involved to rethink their approach to a problem that has been traditionally regarded as a psychological aberration. It is at least possible that the ion effect in man-made environments is a cause of much of the problem—in which case ion depletion and posion poisoning are external forces exerting pressures on our body chemistry. If this is correct, then anxiety should be reclassified as stress; that is, a condition that has a specific and external cause.

However crippling it is, anxiety is hard to describe because its effects are intangible. The F.A.A. scientists who studied the subject came to a similar conclusion about the ion effect. They wrote: "A room that deviates considerably from the optimum ionization condition might not produce an untoward reaction for some time, and when it did the reactions could not be attributed to any directly sensed aspect of the environment. This is perhaps the most frustrating aspect of the study of atmospheric ionization. To acknowledge that an insensible [that is, something one cannot perceive with any of the five senses] factor or agent can exert pervasive effects on one's efficiency or health is almost to admit to belief in the supernatural."

As so many scientists have proved, there is nothing supernatural about the ion effect. It is, in fact, remarkably consistent—and pervasive—and it affects almost every human activity. Take the sad case of the sick sauna, for instance. Historically, the "kiuas," or hearth, of the sauna was made up of preheated stones on which water was poured. Came the Age of Technology and the kiuas was technologized, so that the stones or metal plates on to which water is tossed were heated by electricity. This, of course, is standard in North American saunas, but when it began to creep into the Finnish sauna style five physicists at Tampere

University of Technology in Helsinki grew disturbed and conducted elaborate experiments to measure the effect of electric hearths. They found that when electric stoves were used, great quantities of pos-ions were created, and so instead of being relaxing the electric sauna was producing an element of air electricity that tended to stimulate and even upset the body's chemical balance. The traditional kiuas of preheated stones, however, created massive doses of neg-ions that have a clearly defined tranquilizing effect. When the five physicists published their scientific findings a howl of protest went up throughout Finland, and one traditionalist publicly bemoaned the fact that "the easily regulated, compact, and simple electric heater has, more than anything else, led to the popularity of the Finnish sauna abroad, but also to the decline and degeneration of the Finnish sauna image which we are selling abroad, which now suffers from a moral bankruptcy."

8

"Unhealthy at Any Speed!"

In 1972 three men spent a large part of their working days taking what must have appeared to others to be joy rides through Budapest, out through the suburbs, and into the countryside. Sometimes it was rush hour; sometimes they traveled in the relative quiet of mid-morning. Sometimes it rained; sometimes the sky was leaden, but often it was gloriously sunny and the Danube sparkled as they drove slowly through the city in a variety of ominously official black sedans. Inside the cars the men were relaxed yet watchful, constantly monitoring complex electronic equipment. They, too, were on the trail of the ion effect, only this time they were seeking it in the most common form of transport in the world—the motor vehicle. The aim of the three, all state-employed scientists led by one I. Kerdo, was to find an answer to the question: Is pos-ion poisoning a contributory cause of the increasing road accident rate?

Ion scientists everywhere had long thought that the micro-environment inside motor vehicles was, as one once put it, "inimical to health and safety." They knew that the electrical system of motor vehicles tends to produce pos-ions rather than neg-ions; that car heaters, fresh-air vent systems and air conditioners upset the ionization in much the same way as the duct work of buildings. They knew, too, that in traffic, exhaust fumes produce high concentrations of microscopic particles, and that such dust tends to destroy small, physiologically active ions. All that apart, there is friction between the air and the vehicle as it is moving. This sets up a positive charge on the metal bodywork that acts as a magnet and attracts any neg-ions that may be in the car to the metal. At the same time, of course, this positive charge repels the pos-ions and leaves them to build up in the air inside the car, bus, train, or truck. The conclusion seemed entirely logical: Car drivers get overdoses of pos-ions.

Although in 1965 the Mercedes-Benz company in Germany had embarked on an elaborate series of tests to find out what effect the micro-environment of cars had on drivers and passengers, air electricity had been only one of the elements examined. The Hungarian study was one of the first automotive studies of the ion effect alone. The findings, published the following year, confirmed what police and insurance companies have known for years, that in certain places and at certain times of the year—in southern California during the Santa Ana winds, for instance, or in Jerusalem during the Sharav or in Switzerland and Austria and parts of Germany during the Foehn—the traffic accident rate increases alarmingly. The statistics from most places plagued by Witches' Winds are unreliable but those that are available suggest that, as in Jerusalem during the Sharav, the increase can be more than 100 percent. However, the statistics in Geneva are precise, at least for 1972. In that year, whenever there was a drastic weather change and consequent change in ionization, the accident rate rocketed by over 50 percent. In the most prestigious of all German dictionaries, "Foehn" is partly defined as a meteorological condition that produces reported increases in heart attacks, suicides, and attempted suicides—and in traffic accidents.

There are reasons why the available statistics in this area aren't more detailed. It is impossible to measure the ion count and balance inside a car *after* it has been involved in a pile-up on the New York State Thruway or on the spaghetti of highways in Los Angeles. And even the figures produced by the Hungarians are, scientifically speaking, both inconclusive and suspect since all they do is demonstrate that there is an overdose of pos-ions in motor vehicles. They do not prove that this condition actually causes accidents. The circumstantial evidence to prove that it does is, however, quite impressive.

The Hungarian study was reported in 1973, and in explaining why it was begun, the scientists wrote: "Since the advent of nuclear powered submarines staying submerged for a long time for scientific or strategic reasons, and since the realization of man's space travel, an increasing interest is being shown by scientists in the influence of environmental conditions on human behavior. Conceived in the past to have normally no significant influence on human performance, atmospheric conditions may in fact play a vital role in a small closed space or semi-enclosure. In everyday life a much greater significance is attributed to conditioning the micro-climate of the motor vehicle in such a way that no atmosphere adverse to human performance will be created, thus increasing the safety factor of driving. It cannot be overemphasized that the accomplishment of this latter task will bring closer the solution of a serious, though often subconscious, problem of a large part of mankind. In a closed space the inhalation of even a small percentage of atmospheric contamination for a prolonged period of time will bring about serious biologic consequences leading to a decline in human output. The same applies to changes in the concentration of electrically charged particles floating in that atmosphere, for example, aero-ions. In a majority of cases the crew of a space craft or submarine must work in a totally unnatural ionic atmosphere whose adverse influence may further be enhanced by other factors such as over-strain, by acceleration of stresses, etc. The driver of a car is in a similar condition. The steadily increasing city traffic presents an increasing number of stresses in addition to often raising the carbon dioxide and exhaust gas content of the atmosphere over the permissible level. To make a bad thing worse, meterological influence is often also present in the invasion of warm air masses, producing a prevalence of positive ions. If this influence is superimposed on the adverse conditions of the rush hours, the accident hazard will increase abruptly."

The Hungarian scientists went on to point out that Budapest traffic police statistics proved that when the warm southerly air was present (creating a Foehn condition), the average accident rate increased from a normal peak of 1.6 an hour to 2.6. The tests also demonstrated that even at mid-morning on a winter's day the pos-ion densities in buit-up areas reached what any ion scientist would describe as alarming proportions. Near the Danube and alongside the city parks ionization was low, but the pos-ion to neg-ion ratio was more or less normal. The moment the scientists left the river and park areas and drove through the building-lined streets of the city core, the ratio soared to five pos-ions for every neg-ion. As they drove out through the industrial suburbs and into the country, the ratio went down but inside the urban area it never went below 2.5 to one, in itself an unhealthy ratio.

At the same time this was happening other scientists were studying the micro-climate in trucks, buses, and passenger trains. They concluded that in cities there is an increase in carbon dioxide in the air, and that alone played an important part in increasing the pos-ion dosage. Already heavily dosed with a positive charge, "the air stream flowing through the metal air channels of cooling, heating, and ventilation systems lose electrons upon impacting to the wall or other metal parts, and as a result they are turned into positively charged particles."

The not-surprising result is bad drivers. The Hungarians pointed out that one known effect of pos-ions was the "increased excretion of chemicals associated with tension," while neg-ions tend to have a calming effect. Prof. Gygorgy Adam, also a Hungarian, fed ions to rats in a laboratory and concluded that they learned "defensive" reactions to dangerous situations significantly faster in neg-ion air than in either normal or positively ionized air, and their speed in discriminating between dangerous and safe situations also appeared to increase in air with a neg-ion overdose. Piecing together their own findings and those of other scientists, the three car-driver scientists concluded that the pos-ion overdose inflicted on car drivers everywhere means that "the subject becomes excited and is liable to lose his temper. His movements lose coordination together with a considerable decrease in the concentration of attention. These states have an adverse influence on driving."

Other scientists elsewhere have done work that puts what I consider to be a solid foundation under the wall of circumstantial evidence that pos-ion overdoses cause auto crashes. Sulman in Jerusalem was among the first to prove that people in pos-ion atmospheres did badly when asked to complete a simple intelligence test and that their performance improved in air with a normal ion balance—and improved still further if there was a slight overdose of neg-ions. In the *Journal of Engineering Psychology* in 1965 scientists C. G. Halcomb and R. E. Kirk reported that a group of male university students lost a "very significant" portion of their vigilance after spending three hours in air positively ionized to about the same level as that found in the Hungarian automobiles.

In Hungary the clincher came when the Volan Trust, a group of transportation and manufacturing companies, sent staff psychologists and medical doctors to find out whether truck and bus fleets should be equipped with neg-ion generators. Two hundred professional drivers, one hundred on trucks and the other hundred driving buses, were put through an astonishingly complex series of tests that included spending hours at a time in simulated vehicle cabs facing up to one "driving decision" per second. They were shadowed by driving experts while driving their routes. Their pulse rate, blood pressure, respiration rate, and other bodily functions were measured at the start and the end of a day's driving. And when it was all over the conclusion was that all drivers' performance improved when neg-ion generators were installed near the driver's seat; all drivers were less fatigued and weary at the day's end with an ionizer than they were without one. More significant perhaps was the finding that the performance of those drivers who were weather sensitive deteriorated most rapidly during the day, and improved most noticeably when neg-ion generators were used to restore the ion balance to something approaching normal.

Somewhere in the process of all this research in Budapest, scientists produced an "ion danger-zone" map of the city which showed the areas where pos-ion densities were highest and gave the times of day when the situation was at its worst. From this other scientists have suggested that an additional hazard may be the fact that, in passing through different ion densities and through belts of pollution and weather changes, the driver's body may be subjected to stresses that make him or her even more likely to be an accident looking for a place to happen.

Discovering the research material relating to cars and driving was disconcerting to me, since it suggests that as a weather sensitive person I am likely to be a less capable driver than most. Most people drive sedans or station wagons and on touring holidays the driver is at the wheel for as much as six to eight hours at a time. The pos-ion concentration in cars may conveniently explain cranky kids and rows between husband and wife, but it also represents a threat to driver, passengers, and to other road users everywhere and at all times.

Since the time of the Hungarian research into the ion effect in motor vehicles, several European auto makers have shown an interest in the subject. Mercedes-Benz in Germany was a pioneer in this field, and their conclusions that the micro-environment in cars had a damaging effect on drivers' abilities and comfort leave one wondering why no car maker has yet installed corrective devices. Perhaps the reason is that production technology always lags years behind the original scientific development; after all, it took a quarter century to get the Wankel rotary engine to the new car showrooms. In the meantime several European motorists' organizations have issued warnings about the perils of pos-ion poisoning in cars. The Touring Club Suisse reports the traffic accident increase during the Foehn, and typically the British Automobile Association's recent publication, *The Book of the Car*, says: "Stuffiness inside a car leads to lethargy and a loss of concentration. A disadvantage of the modern car's heating-ventilation system is that it upsets the electrical balance of the fresh air it supplies. Electrically charged particles, or ions, in the atmosphere affect the way we feel or act. Too many negatively charged ions in the atmosphere or at high altitudes leads to a feeling of exhilaration. Too many positively charged ions, as before a storm, induce drowsiness and depression. The proportion of positive ions in the air is increased when the air is drawn through a car heater. Opening a side window freshens the air inside the vehicle by restoring the balance between positive and negative ions." While it is not entirely scientifically accurate this kind of comment in authoritative drivers' manuals throughout Europe has prompted many drivers to acquire small neg-ion generators that plug into the dashboard cigarette lighter. North American drivers are less likely to open windows than most; Detroit stopped building convertibles several years ago, and about 13 percent of American cars—that is, 1,300,000 or thereabouts in the 1975–76 model year —are sold with air conditioners as well as heaters.

But what of other forms of transportation? Planes, for instance? Because of the jobs I've held in the management of several multinational corporations, I

have flown a great deal, and have often found the behavior of people on planes quite fascinating. Flying
makes many anxious and tense, but some people can
instantly fall asleep. I usually do. Others are stimulated and excited and appear to drink a great deal
more than I should think would be normal for most
people without a drinking problem. There are, of
course, many possible explanations. Some of us worry
about the safety of the plane; others have flown so
often they are blasé and simply regard flight time as a
useful rest period between hectic meetings. Others are
excited at their prospects upon arrival. However,
such passenger behavior could be explained by the
ion effect—and there are ion scientists who say that it
is the lack of neg-ions and the preponderance of pos-
ions that cause the varied reactions of plane passengers, and may also be a contributory cause to many
air crashes.

The principle involved in aircraft pressurization
is so similar to that of other artificial air treatment
systems that in airplanes, as in air-conditioned offices
and cars, the healthy balance between pos-ions and
neg-ions is totally destroyed. Rosemary Dudley, who
abandoned an active career as a writer to become
head of the Migraine Foundation in Canada, has told
me that migraine victims frequently suffer agonies as a
plane either takes off or lands and the air pressure
and humidity change slightly in the cabin. But she also
says that others—perhaps those who suffer from Horton's Migraine that Dr. Fox successfully treated with
neg-ion generators in England—may suffer a violent attack in a normal flight for no apparent reason.

The F.A.A. researchers concluded that the ion
threshold below which pos-ions could begin to have
a detrimental effect on human performance and comfort was 1,000 ions per cubic centimeter, of which
two-thirds are pos-ions and only one-third neg-ions.
Apart from the fact that by this rather arbitrary
definition, no apartment or office block is healthy, it
is also probable that ionization in aircraft cabins and
cockpits is below this threshold. The likely explanation

is that the friction generated on the outer skin of the plane generates a massive positive charge, and that any neg-ions left in the air inside are drawn to the body of the plane. The situation is probably less serious in the passenger cabin, where the outer metalwork is partly insulated with decorative plastic panels, but could be bad on the flight deck, where there is a great deal of exposed metal to act as magnets to what neg-ions there are in the air. I know of no published reports of research done on aircraft in flight, and none was reported by the F.A.A. researchers, but they did say, "Ionization of the atmosphere in aircraft may be an important factor in the health and comfort of passengers in commercial aviation and general aviation pilots. An atmosphere that is predominantly negatively ionized, that contains an excess of negative ions, improves the process of oxygenation of the blood, and excessive positive ions may interfere with the oxygenation of the blood."

Ionization is an element in the argument of Florida doctor-cum-jet pilot E. Stanton Maxey, who says that in certain conditions the electrical balance on flight decks is a potential cause of crashes. In April 1973 he wrote to the New York Times: "Last December 29 almost 100 New York passengers bought death tickets aboard Eastern Airlines Flight 401. That Lockheed 1011 cost about $15 million. Litigation will range in hundreds of millions. Might a $500 gadget have kept all safe? Since Eastern's pilots Robert Loft and Albert Stockstill failed to react to altimeters, pilot error becomes obvious. The flight recorder heard the audible alarm at 1,700 feet but neither pilot responded. Crew member Angelo Donadel survived to report 'there was never any alarm or concern in the cockpit.' Picture it: A $15 million jet is flying into the ground and two superb pilots simultaneously quit seeing and hearing instruments. They are not even concerned. Were both pilots slipped an electrical mickey?"

As we shall see later, Maxey is not suggesting that ionization is the only problem in such circumstances, and he makes it clear that the atmospheric conditions that existed at the time of the crash of Flight 401 are so rare as to be almost unique. On the other hand, there is clear laboratory evidence from scientists both in North America and the rest of the world that upsetting the ion count and balance causes, at the very least, a lack of vigilance and a slowing in reaction time, both perilous when a pilot is trying to safely land an airborne behemoth.

In his book *Human Factors in Air Transportation: Occupational and Health Safety,* R. A. MacFarland suggests that the old rule that "those who can walk may fly" should be revised. He says that those suffering from a variety of noncrippling diseases should, in fact, avoid air travel. He lists heart disease, angina, anemia, emphysema, asthma, pneumonia, and diabetes. It is worth remembering that in the Foehn, the Sharav, and in laboratory tests all these conditions (with the exception of diabetes) have been shown to be susceptible to the ion effect. That dictionary definition of the Foehn I mentioned earlier makes it clear that one consequence of that particular Witches' Wind is heart and circulation problems. And all respiratory problems are inflamed if there is a high overdose of pos-ions. The F.A.A. researchers, after rejecting a suggestion that the ion levels in aircraft represented a danger, ended their report by saying: "In the light of the concern over environmental quality and with the knowledge of the demonstrated effects of atmospheric ions, it would appear appropriate at this time to conduct a survey of existing levels of atmospheric ionization in the passenger cabins and cockpits of commercial flights at cruising altitudes." This report was completed in 1972. I am not aware that any such survey has yet been conducted.

In a sense cars, buses, trains, and airplanes are, along with heated and cooled buildings and other elements of any urban environment, what Henry L. Logan, a New York lighting engineer, has called the "clothing" that has made man's progress possible. Logan's argument is that wherever it was that man first evolved as something superior to the apes, he would never have been able to take over the world without clothing, some covering that enabled him to survive in other environments. Logan argues that by this definition housing and all forms of transportation are manmade environments that can be called clothing. He says that until this century all such clothing was of natural materials, but that because of the technological revolution this clothing is now created out of unnatural materials in unnatural circumstances. "The technological age of the twentieth century presents the first total threat to man because it changes the rules of survival as he has known them up to now by changing his immediate environment," says Logan.

It is a persuasive argument, but ironically Logan's use of the word clothing is more significant than perhaps even he realizes. We are now wearing clothes—pants, dresses, shirts, blouses, underwear—that are made of unnatural, or synthetic, materials, and clearly do change the rules of survival because they change the most immediate environment of all—that on and near the surface of the skin.

Almost everyone has experienced a mild electric shock when, in dry weather, he or she walks briskly through home or office and then touches a piece of metal—an elevator button, perhaps, or a typewriter or doorknob. Everyone knows this is caused by static electricity; that static is a charge that builds up on the body as a result of friction as one walks; that walking on broadloom is the most common way in which this friction is caused. And yet it can happen when there is no carpet. Why? Because almost everyone wears clothes that are totally or partly made from synthetic fabrics. And the most commonly used synthetic fabrics have what is called a positive potential—that is, when rubbed they generate a positive charge that causes clothing to cling to the body and sparks to fly when you undress.

Thus our clothing is an outer "skin" that carries an active electrical charge. If this second skin has a positive charge, it tends to attract the neg-ions in the air we breathe to the clothing, thus diminishing the number available for inhalation. Our skin also absorbs some of the charge generated by clothing, so that if that charge is positive the neg-ions in the air we breathe are attracted to the positively charged skin of our faces, and the air we actually inhale contains fewer neg-ions than it otherwise would. On the other hand, those synthetic fabrics that can create a negative static charge will repel the neg-ions—drive them out of the air immediately around us. They also, of course, attract pos-ions.

Most of us are totally unaware of any effect, but asthmatics or people with emphysema and other respiratory ills often suffer additional agonies because of the clothes they wear, and are just as often unaware of the reason why they suffer. Dr. Bernard Watson, professor of medical electronics at Britain's St. Bartholomew's Teaching Hospital in London, says: "Changing the immediate unhealthy ion environment to help an asthmatic means changing everything, clothes, sheets, furniture—just everything." When we talked in London he also told me of one patient, a girl at that time fourteen, who had begun to suffer from severe migraine because of clothing—and then cured it herself. When she grew to adolescence and began to wear, with great pride, nylon bras and panties favored by most women, she began to suffer from occasional headaches for the first time in her life. When she graduated to slips and nightdresses and pretty nylon blouses, she became a full-fledged migraine sufferer. Her local general practitioner could offer neither explanation nor help beyond suggesting the onset of menstruation as a cause. But the girl was bright enough to associate the clothes of blooming womanhood with her problem and promptly abandoned the feminine underwear and nightdresses. Now her clothes are of cotton, which is the only fiber that creates no charge at all, and of natural fibers like wool, which carry little charge of either kind. However, once migraine has taken root it is not easy to cure and Dr. Watson is still treating the girl, in part by suggesting to her parents that certain items of furniture in their home should be removed.

The issue of furniture—of the materials with which we surround ourselves—is awesomely complex. Generally speaking, however, it may be said that synthetic materials in all furnishings—carpets, chairs, sofas, tables, curtains—upset the ion balance. In all but the 25 to 30 percent of cases where people are weather sensitive, the effect may not be so noticeable that it is troublesome. At the International Ion Research Congress in Philadelphia in 1961, C. W. Hansell, the ion scientist from the R.C.A. research laboratories, said: "Our distant ancestors in the course of our evolutionary development lived literally with their feet on the ground. Their bodies were kept at ground potential. In contrast, we are electrically insulated from the ground for much of the time, often with our bodies at potentials far different from ground and our surroundings. These potentials can have large effects upon the ratio of positive to negative ions we absorb from the air and upon their total number. An outstanding example is provided in warm dry air in winter when we walk about on clean, new wool carpets in rubber- or leather-soled shoes. Our bodies may then become negatively charged to potentials of tens of thousands of volts. Under these circumstances negative ions are strongly repelled by our negatively charged bodies but positive ions are strongly attracted. We are then likely to be physically, mentally, and emotionally depressed and irritable."

Christian Bach, a Danish pioneer in ion science (an electrical engineer, he began his research in 1953) tells how he suffered from asthma until he built a simple ionizer from designs published in the American magazine *Science Digest*. In the years since he has become an acknowledged authority on what he calls the "passive therapy" approach in which he studies the clothing and environment of asthmatics and others who suffer from pos-ion poisoning, then pinpoints the offending fabrics and articles that are throwing the ion effect out of balance.

What is intriguing is that early on Bach discovered what scientists were to prove later—that plants are nature's most prolific source of neg-ions since they conduct the negative energy of the earth up into the air and "eject" it from the tips of their leaves. Early in what were at first rather unscientific experiments he used asparagus plants growing in an electrical field to generate neg-ions. Judging from reports in his book *Ions for Breathing*, published in England in 1967, the plants seem to have worked well.

In reporting the work of the Danish Air Ionization Institute, of which he is director, Bach says that he and his colleagues have worked with many hospitals in treating victims of asthma and other respiratory ills. He tells what has become a classic case history involving a woman who had asthma in her own apartment but not in the homes of friends. Even a neg-ion generator was of no help, so Bach conducted what must have been one of the oddest investigations in history: Was the culprit the furniture, the television set, the bedding, the lamp shades? Bach found that the lady's taste ran mostly to modern synthetic fabrics. However, that alone was insufficient to explain the problem, so eventually Bach began cross-examining the woman about her housekeeping. He found that her furniture was treated with cellulose- and silicone-based furniture finishes. Laboratory tests proved that such finishes, when rubbed with polishing rags and dusters, produce a positive charge. Then he visited the friends in whose home her asthma condition disappeared. There he found that the furniture was hand polished with old-fashioned wax and elbow grease, which produced no static charge at all. Bach coated the victim's furniture with an antistatic compound, told her to buy antique furniture without modern wood treatments, and her asthma attacks ceased.

In all, Bach had by 1967 treated almost 1,000 hay fever and asthma cases whose problems were cured or eased by his "passive therapy" approach. In one case, he says, a man became an asthma victim because his wife bought two new lamp shades that led to the overproduction of positive ions; in another instance several members of the same family became sufferers because their new television set had a teak cabinet that had been treated with cellulose. He also tells of one instance in which he was called in to help save the fortunes of chicken farmer Flemming Juncker in the town of Overgard. Farmer Juncker had two monstrous chicken houses each housing 20,000 chickens. In one of them, between 150 and 200 chickens died every week. Bach found that both chicken houses were of identical design and construction, except that the one where the chickens died had a roof lined with sheets of plastic while the other building had a roof of wood. Whenever there was a change in the weather the death rate went up. Bach concluded that when weather changes affected air electricity the plastic stimulated the production of pos-ion overdoses. He treated the roof with an antistatic substance, and within weeks the chicken mortality rate was normal in both hen coops.

Perhaps without realizing it, Dr. Watson in London and others who, disregarding the controversy over the ion effect, use it as a practical therapy for the victims of many ailments are commonly using variations of Christian Bach's "passive therapy." Bach himself suggests that the reason why the Danes are ahead of the world in their awareness of the effects of clothing and furniture is because Denmark has more air conditioning and central heating than most nations. And, he argues, the Danes are world leaders in using new materials for furniture designs—materials that, because they are generally synthetic, can make life miserable for those among us who are acutely ion sensitive.

Like all Scandinavians, the Danes keep their homes spotless, forever flourishing dusters, wielding brooms, pushing vacuum cleaners, and otherwise raising clouds of dust to which neg-ions are attracted, and so disappear as physiologically active small ions. It is, it would seem, healthier to be a sloppy housewife than a meticulous one. At that International Ion Research

Conference in Philadelphia in 1961, Dr. Hansell ended his speech by saying that to prevent a buildup of potentially harmful ions the husband who comes home from work should promptly take his shoes off and walk around the carpets in his stockinged feet. And he added, "My suggestion to the wives is that it is a very well known fact that it is very difficult to get a charge from a dirty surface. They should not, I suggest, be too houseproud."

9

Ions and Sex

As I have already confessed, one of the effects of my Geneva "condition" was the dramatic diminishing of my sex drive. To find that in my early thirties and usually in the spring I often lost much of my zest and enthusiasm for the fundamental relationship between man and woman was perhaps the most disturbing single symptom of all. After I learned from Dr. Wissmer—the man who first suggested there was "something electrical" about the air in Geneva—that I was just one of many Foehn victims, I realized that my sex drive diminished only at the time of the Foehn. I also began to wonder to what degree the ion effect plays a part in personal relationships. Along with Masters and Johnson and a great many sex therapists, I have long believed in the truth of the old saying: "If the bedroom isn't happy, then neither is any room in the house." I belong to that generation which, buffeted by an abandonment of old moralities and a bewildering rate of change of all kinds, sometimes seems incapable of making the tranditional husband-and-wife living arrangement work. Like most fairly successful and affluent men of my age, I find most of my friends and colleagues have already parted from their first wives or say privately that they are unhappily married. And one of the most common complaints I hear from both men and women is that in their marriages their sex lives either were or are unsatisfying. There are many possible explanations, not the least of them being a new frankness about sex and, because of the liberation movement, a new awareness among women of their own sexual potential along with a demand that it be fulfilled. Even so, can what appears to be a widespread dissatisfaction be linked to what I discovered about the unhealthy ion levels and balances in the urban world in which most of us live?

Clearly the ion levels in the air must have an effect on the lives of those of us who are acutely ion sensitive. If you've got an asthma attack or a migraine, you aren't likely to feel sexy as well. If you just feel below par, unhappy, tense, and anxious—and perhaps worried because there is no rational explanation for these feelings—then, whether man or woman, you are not likely to be much fun in bed. Survival is the most fundamental instinct of all, and if your health appears to be bad the second most powerful drive—the sex urge—is the most noticeable thing to suffer. From Dr. Wissmer, I learned that there were many people in Geneva so afflicted, although he pointed out that many of them, acting almost in panic, actively sought relationships outside their marriages because a new romance revived their flagging interest in sex, at least for a while. In my own case, I always found that my sex drive revived whenever I left Geneva, although I am frankly still not certain how much of that was due to the stimulus of new surroundings and people and how much had to do with finding myself in a healthier ion environment.

But surely some of this argument can apply to almost everyone. After all, although 25 percent of the population appears not to suffer at all when the ion environment is upset, that still leaves 75 percent of all humans who are more or less affected even if they don't suffer as we ion sensitives, or weather sensitives, do. If a man or woman living in an urban atmosphere that is generally ion depleted also spends a day at work in a heated or air-conditioned building where the massive ion depletion and pos-ion poisoning are so much worse, then he or she ends the day tired and irritable and generally out of sorts. That person is not likely to be either sexually stimulating or stimulated. A person who has spent all his or her bodily vitality coping with the environment at work is not likely to have much energy left over for the bedroom.

One quite beautiful woman I know in Zurich once told me in a moment of disconcerting frankness that the Foehn left her feeling so uninterested in sex that, on Foehn days, she always carefully arranged things so her husband would go to bed first. Then she would go to the bathroom and wait behind the door until she heard him begin to snore. "Sometimes he wakes up early in the morning though, and then I just grin and bear it," she said. "I don't want to become one of those wives who's always pleading a headache, but in the Foehn I sympathize with them. All my energy is sapped and I feel so below par that it's about all I can do to keep myself alive from one end of the day to the other." One can never be sure about such things but, Foehn apart, I would be ready to swear that that particular couple probably enjoys one of the healthiest and most energetic relationships imaginable.

Once I tracked down and questioned a building supply sales manager who lived near Lugano and whose firm had six months earlier equipped all its offices with table-top neg-ion generators. I simply wanted to ask what effects, if any, he had noticed since the equipment had been installed. He was a quiet and thoughtful man, by no means the hearty, extroverted salesman type, and I was therefore the more astonished when he instantly replied: "Well, the biggest effect has been on my sex life; my wife loves it." He went on to explain that after the ionizer had been installed he felt more alert and energetic at work and, since he spent part of each week driving to see clients, he had then installed a smaller ionizer in his car. Soon afterward he installed one at home in his bedroom. "I'm not saying it does anything to me physically, but it certainly gives me more energy. I used to go home quite played out, too tired to do anything much but eat and sit and stare at television. But now I seem to have lots of energy left. We go out more, and my wife enjoys that, and I'm not so tired when we go to bed and . . . well, as I said, it has done a lot for my sex life and that means it helps my marriage as well."

From all this one can easily conclude that unhealthy ionization may at the very least have some secondhand effect on our sex lives because the illnesses and conditions directly caused by pos-ion poisoning are likely to make us less interested in the subject. But there is a great deal of evidence to suggest that pos-ion overdoses also affect the parts of the body that are directly involved in sexual activity.

One of Dr. Albert Krueger's early experiments involved silk worms. He found that in certain concentrations of either ion the larvae matured into adults earlier, and that the adults mated earlier than usual. I won't use the specific measurements, since they are bewilderingly scientific, but ions did increase the rate of growth of the larvae. The silk worms also produced much richer and more luxuriant cocoons of silk, a laboratory finding that has been put to good commercial use in Japan, where neg-ion generators are used in silk farms to make silk worms "sexy."

R. Gualtierotti, the director of the Research Center of Medical Bioclimatology at the University of Milan, conducted experiments with mice, and one result was that both males and females matured very rapidly in negatively ionized air. When mature, the female mice were much more fecund than normal. He subsequently wrote in the *Aeroionotherapy Journal,* published by the prestigious Carlo Erba Foundation: "Many authors have noted an increase in sexual activity in man as a result of exposure to aeroions. This has been confirmed by a series of experiments on animals living in an environment of artificially negatively ionized air. Histological examination of testicles and ovaries of animals exposed to high concentrations of negative ions for ninety-six hours shows a definite stimulation of the process of maturation of a large number of cells." More simply put, Gualtierotti believes that a preponderance of neg-ions stimulates sexual activity and tends to make men more fertile and women more fecund.

The fact that neg-ions have a massive effect on the testicles of animals probably has some bearing on the two main sexual problems reported by men—premature ejaculation and occasional impotence. If neg-ions stimulate the activity of our sexual organs, then it is likely that pos-ion poisoning may have the reverse effect.

In women, the reproductive organs are demonstrably affected by ions. We have already seen that the full moon produces an increase in positive ionization, and at the same time seems to induce the birth of the baby if the pregnancy is about ended. But Felix Sulman in Jerusalem has demonstrated a more direct link between ions, the production of serotonin, and the female reproductive organs.

Dr. Sulman's work as an ion scientist began because the university hospital's department of gynecology wanted to study the effect of serotonin in childbirth; it was only later that he found that serotonin production was stimulated by pos-ions. One of Sulman's first steps was to try to find out what role serotonin played in the bodies of women known as "habitual aborters"—that is, women who have repeatedly tried and failed to carry a baby for a full nine months. First he experimented on rats, and found that pregnant rats aborted if injected with serotonin. Then twenty women who sought and were given permission to have legal abortions were given drugs that artificially caused their bodies to produce an overdose of serotonin. In each case this serotonin overproduction caused an abortion. Having found that the neurohormone could cause abortions, Dr. Sulman theorized that perhaps it was the cause of continual abortions in women who actually wanted children. So in the late 1950s and early 1960s he treated more than one hundred "habitual aborters" with drugs that blocked, or prevented, the natural serotonin production process. It worked. Almost all the women who had repeatedly tried and failed to become mothers gave birth to healthy infants.

The serotonin overproduction was only occasionally caused by pos-ion poisoning due to the Sharav. In most cases there was no obvious external explanation for the fact that the women's bodies simply produced more serotonin than their reproductive systems could handle. In others, the stress involved in trying to have babies and fearing failure may in itself have been enough to cause overproduction of serotonin; it is, after all, a stress neurohormone. In one otherwise very formal scientific paper, Sulman reported: "We encountered twelve cases where the regimen of daily urine collection [to test the serotonin content] was sufficient in itself to prevent recurring serotonin abortion. The reason for this unexpected success was the avoidance of friction with the family, especially with the husband. When a querulous husband who disapproved of the pregnancy was kept busy collecting his wife's urine, measuring it, labeling it, and transferring it to a laboratory, he identified himself with the problems of the wife, and, participating in her distress, contributed decisively to the disappearance of high serotonin levels."

After treating "habitual aborters" for almost a decade, new regulations in Israel forbade the use of the specific serotonin-blocking drug Dr. Sulman had used in pregnancy cases with such success. However, during one of my recent visits to Israel, he told me with quiet pride one evening: "We have more than a hundred serotonin children and babies in this country that would never have been born if we hadn't done what we did."

Breasts aren't directly involved in the reproductive process, but they are very much part of our sex lives —and they are affected by ions. As long ago as 1927 an Italian scientist, L. M. Spolverini, reported that ionization caused a "remarkable" increase in the milk secretion in both women and animals who had just given birth. More recently, Russian ion scientists treating new mothers with neg-ions to help them recover from the effects of having just given birth were told by the women themselves that the neg-ions helped them give milk to their offspring. The doctors promptly mounted a systematic study of the effect of neg-ions on lactation in women and found that those who normally had a generous supply of milk were not much affected, but women who had been unable to feed their babies prior to neg-ion therapy were able to do so quite happily afterward. As in all the research into the ion effect, the Russian finding was that neg-ions had a distinct value as a medical therapy in cases of physiological abnormality, but little effect on normal and healthy people —and no harmful effects on anyone, whether sick or not.

In the 1950s a British statesman introduced new laws that would remove most so-called sexual offenses from the criminal code with the now immortal phrase, "The state has no place in the bedrooms of the nation." Neither have I, or rather, neither have my comments. But perhaps a neg-ion generator does have such a place. It may be worth remembering, however, that the scientific literature includes the reported case of a man of ninety who took a new young wife to a spa in Yugoslavia where the neg-ion count is very high—and within the first week sired his twenty-first child.

10

Our Bioelectric World

The ion effect is not the only electrical phenomenon vital to life on earth. The energy from the ionosphere, the sun and moon, and from the earth's surface not only produces ions, but also creates an electrical field that is a different but closely related phenomenon. If I may be forgiven a necessary but not entirely scientific simplification, the ions are "active" in that they carry a specific charge, while the electrical field is "passive" because it doesn't. Since the field, too, is part of the environment, it must also have a profound effect on all living matter, although right now science knows precious little about what those effects might be. One thing we do know, however, is that the field has in it waves of extremely low frequencies (a maximum of around 100 cycles per second, compared with 500,000 cps for the lowest commercial radio frequency) and that right at the bottom of this so-called ELF (extremely low frequency) range are the wavelengths on which the human brain functions. When asleep, our brain activity can be measured at between 5 and 7 cycles per second; when awake it is between 10 and 15 cps. Dr. Walter Stark, one of many ion scientists who have be-

gun studying electric field effects, says that the waves
in this field "serve as a sort of pacemaker to the
brain." Since this seems likely, it is also at least possible that variations and distortions in the field may
affect human beings.

'   The ion scientists' interest in electrical fields was
aroused by awareness of the fact that artificially generated electrical fields—those set up by an electrical
appliance, for instance—influence the ion effect, a subject I shall discuss later. They reason that if man-
made electrical fields can influence ion counts and
balances, then so can variations in the electrical field
caused by weather and perhaps by the radioactive content of the soil and rock strata in a particular area.
Thus men of the stature of Dr. Stark, Dr. Krueger, and
Dr. Sulman consider the subject a logical next step in
their ion research.

Perhaps the most dramatic evidence that the
health and efficiency of humans must be affected by all
forms of air electricity is Kirlian photography, a technique imported from the U.S.S.R. that actually photographs the electrical "aura" that surrounds all living
things. It works simply. You place your fingers on a
piece of sensitized paper laid over a copper plate
through which a low charge of electricity is passed.
When developed by normal photographic processes,
the paper produces a picture of the strength of the
bioelectrical energy—or aura—streaming from your
fingers. It is also possible to take such photographs of
many parts of the body, and some doctors believe they
have learned how to diagnose your physical and mental health from the appearance of this aura. Perhaps the
best-known Kirlian photography experiments involve
leaves plucked from trees. Photographs taken hours
apart show how the amount of bioelectricity in the
leaves diminishes as they die. When humans are sick,
the amount of this electrical energy available to be pho-
tographed diminishes. The aura "fades."

As I have said, the earth's electrical field can be
distorted by local weather conditions, and this may explain why in Switzerland and southern Germany the

word "Foehn" is used not only to describe a wind, but also to describe a "condition" that often exists even when the wind is not blowing. Had I suffered in Geneva only on those days when the wind blew I would probably never have grown so concerned that I would have embarked on my "Ion Odyssey." In fact, however, my problems beset me even when the wind itself was not blowing, and they did so because of this "Foehn condition."

Geneva lies at the end of the lake of the same name, where two mountain ranges converge to form a V-shaped funnel. The city itself is to the north of these mountains. The Foehn blows from the southeast, flying up over the mountains and falling into the valley in which both city and lake are located. It is trapped there by thermal inversion, that is, the Foehn air is warm but the upper layers of air are cold and the two don't mix. Thus the Foehn air, massively overloaded with pos-ions, is trapped at ground level over the city. A similar inversion can take place on warm days in most cities; the air close to the ground warms up because paved streets, buildings, and pollution store the sun's energy. In the case of Geneva, however, the city is in the point of the V and is sheltered from other winds and breezes. Thus the Foehn air stays in place longer than it does just a few miles away, up the lake. Dr. Stark believes this already bad situation is worsened by electrical activity between the layers of warm and cold air that make up the thermal inversion. Such activity, he says, produces local electrical disturbances and these in turn may influence the ion effect in the air in which the people of Geneva are bathed. The precise mechanism has yet to be explained, but the result is that the Foehn condition persists long after the Foehn wind has blown itself out.

A similar situation exists in many parts of Switzerland, Austria, and southern Germany, and while no one can fully explain the why and how of it, the Swiss Meteorologist Institute in its report, "Foehn and Weather Sensitiveness," draws a distinction between the Foehn wind and the far more frequent Foehn condition. For instance, such a condition often exists when Geneva is swept by its other prevailing wind, the Bise, that blusters out of the north and bounces off the mountains, turning back on itself to fall on the city. Just a few miles up the lake the wind is still troublesome, but the Foehn condition is rarely experienced: In Lausanne, for instance, barely thirty miles away, the climate is acknowledged to be far healthier than in Geneva, probably due to the fact that the city is built in an open area that is exposed to other winds and breezes, which constantly clear the air. Many other parts of Switzerland are not so fortunate; they are so plagued by both Foehn wind *and* Foehn condition that the Swiss Meteorological Institute is often asked to recommend Foehn-free areas of the country by people who are particularly weather sensitive and want to move to end their agonies. The Institute reports that those who seek to escape both the wind and the condition report similar complaints and problems to those which I suffered in Geneva and which are reported in the Sharav areas of Israel, the Sirocco of Italy, the Mistral of France, and the Santa Ana of California.

The Institute found that even in the Foehn condition there was an excess of pos-ions, and it conceded that meteorologists are often unable to explain why some larger cities, individual neighborhoods, and even specific streets have earned local reputations as "Foehn holes." Even in the same city there are apparently remarkable differences in the atmospheric electrical field and, since the Institute recommended neg-ion machines "to bring on the missing negative ions," it may be presumed that "Foehn holes" are places where there is an unhealthy overdose of pos-ions. While meteorologists may be puzzled, ion scientists have an explanation for this phenomenon. They argue that a city that, in theory, should be particularly unhealthy may in fact not be so because of the land on which it is built. For instance, by all the rules of ion science New York streets should be so overloaded with positive electrical charge that an ion-sensitive person like me should find the place at best exhausting. It is one of the paradoxes of the effects of air electricity that I do not find it so; rather the reverse is true.

In 1972 I accompanied Dr. Stark on a walk through the concrete canyons of Manhattan where, with a portable ion counter, he measured the ion density and balance. We found only a few hundred ions at sidewalk level, and almost all of those were posions. Dr. Stark's belief is that in some yet unexplained way the rock strata on which New York is built affects the natural electrical field and to some extent counteracts what would otherwise be an unhealthy situation in the streets and open spaces of New York. This argument does not, however, apply to the hermetically sealed office buildings, hotels, stores, and apartment houses that cover Manhattan Island.

If, in fact, the Foehn condition is largely due to disturbances in the natural electrical field rather than to direct changes in ion count and balance, then the subject merits more and urgent investigation. That Swiss Meteorological Institute report is one of the most recent and comprehensive documents on the effect of weather and environment on human beings. It was published in 1974, and the list of physical and mental ills that it said are caused by both the Foehn wind and the condition is terrifying.

"Physical: Body pains, sick headaches, dizziness, twitching of the eyes, nausea, fatigue, faintness, disorders in saline (salt) budget with fluctuations in electrolytical metabolism (calcium, magnesium; critical for alcoholics), water accumulation, respiratory difficulties, allergies, asthma, heart and circulatory disorders (heart attacks approximately 50 percent higher in Munich), low blood pressure or drop in blood pressure, slowing down in reaction time, more sensitivity to pain, inflammations, bleeding, embolisms of the lungs, and thrombosis.

"Psychological: Emotional unbalance, irritation, vital disinclination, compulsion to meditate, exhaustion, apathy, disinclination or listlessness toward work (poor school achievement), insecurity, anxiety, depression (especially after age forty to fifty); rate of attempted suicide about 20 percent higher, larger number of admittances to clinics in drug cases."

From all the findings of ion science it is clear that those of us who are ion sensitive are more likely to produce overdoses of serotonin in our bodies and this explains most, if not all of our problems. Why we should suffer more than others of the species is not yet known, but reports at a conference of scientists held in 1976 at the University of California at Davis provides some clues. More than 400 evolutionists, geneticists, and biochemists from around the world attended that conference with the aim of relating scientific discoveries made in the previous ten years to Darwin's theory of evolution. At that conference the true bioelectric nature of living organisms became more apparent than ever before.

A case in point was the discussion of the new discoveries about proteins. Proteins are simply long chains of amino acids, but they exist in a bewildering variety and carry out all the processes of creating and sustaining life. In the past decade scientists had for the first time conducted experiments that involved placing proteins in electrical fields. They found that the proteins were drawn either to the negative or the positive sides of the field, indicating that they had a negative or positive potential. When several proteins were placed in a field, each of them behaved differently; each moved at a different rate toward the two polarities. The conclusion was that each protein had its own "electro-signature."

This itself didn't shake the common belief that the same protein—say, one from the hemoglobin molecule of blood—from two human beings would always be the same, would always have the same electro-signature. But then scientists did take identical proteins from two human beings—and found that they, too, behaved differently when placed in an electrical field. Each had a totally different signature. Until that experiment we had all believed that people are different because of heredity or personality or glands. However, as the conference organizer, Dr. Francisco

Ayala, said, "Contrary to popular belief, this new technique shows there is an extraordinary diversity among individuals at the biochemical level."

All this lends a new dimension to Darwin's theory of the survival of the fittest, namely, we must also be biochemically fit to survive changes in the earth's electrical fields. Perhaps the most tragic example of those who are clearly unfit to survive by this definition is the mentally unbalanced. In the early 1960s three New York State professors—Howard Friedman of Syracuse Veterans Administration Hospital, Charles H. Bachman of Syracuse University, and Robert O. Becker of the State University of New York—related the admission rate at seven state psychiatric hospitals to changes in the electrical field in the area. The study lasted from July 1, 1957 to October 31, 1961. In the famous scientific magazine *Nature* the three scientists later wrote that "a significant relationship has been shown between psychiatric disturbance as reflected in hospital admissions" and natural field intensity. How many New Yorkers in that time had psychological or emotional upsets and either never bothered or couldn't afford to seek professional help?

Robert Becker persisted in this area of research and by December 1972 was writing in the *Massachusetts Institute of Technology Review* that: "We are on the threshold of a new era in medicine in which bioelectronics offers the clinician control over basic life processes which even a decade ago could not have been anticipated." When he wrote that, he had in mind not only our bodily health but our mental equilibrium. Psychiatrists have long talked of a suicide belt in Central Europe, encompassing Hungary, Austria, Switzerland, and Bavaria. And the suicide rate is at its highest during the Foehn condition in all those countries, just as it soars during the Santa Ana in California, along with the accident rate, the heart attack rate, and the incidence of apparently pointless crimes of violence.

Electrical fields may also have both political and sociological significance. Walter Stark and several other scientists have suggested that local variations in the electrical field and in ionization may help explain differences in national characteristics. From experience I can testify that to survive in Geneva one needs to develop a phlegmatic and self-disciplined approach to life—a self-imposed regimen of thought and behavior that enables one to stay in control of the effects of pos-ion poisoning. The Swiss of Geneva—indeed, the Swiss generally—have developed such a regimen as part of their social structure and national character. What everyone says about the Swiss is true—they are a diligent and hard-working nation, but they are rather joyless. There may even be a significant connection between the fact that Calvin was born and lived in Geneva, and that Calvinism is a dour, joyless, self-disciplined form of Christian worship.

Stark also suggests that the Sharav that plagues Israel, particularly Jerusalem, may have had a major influence on the character of the Jewish people. He argues that when they were slaves of the Egyptians, the Jews were a docile, tractable people, but after Moses led them to the Sharav-swept Promised Land they became rebellious and hard to govern, as the Romans found at considerable cost. The people of Foehn-swept southern Germany—Bavaria—have also had a reputation in history as rebellious, stubborn, and independent. The Roman Emperor Claudius is reported to have once said of the people of what we now know as southern Germany: "They seem to be an exceptionally nervous and quarrelsome people." Rather more recently, the Belgian researcher Yves F. Pajot wrote: "Many irrational attitudes encountered in the Middle East could be directly or indirectly attributed to mental disturbances provoked by frequent exposures to abnormally high positive ion concentrations." It's certainly true that the Jews of Israel are not the only stubborn people in that part of the world; in the past twenty years a half dozen or more alliances of the Arab states have fallen apart over issues that elsewhere in the world might have been settled by a little stiff-lipped diplomacy. I report all this without comment, since I would rather not take the seductive route of blaming all my personal shortcomings on the place where I was born (Czechoslovakia) or the land where I grew up (North America).

E. Stanton Maxey, the Florida physician and jet pilot whom I have previously mentioned, has suggested that Eastern Airlines Flight 401 to Florida in December 1972, may have crashed because its "two superb pilots" were affected by changes in the force field in the cockpit. It is a speculative argument, but perhaps worth considering in view of the fact that humans did evolve to function in a certain low-strength electrical field, and may possibly be affected by sudden fluctuations in that field.

Maxey pointed out that the plane was landing in an area where electrical storms and disturbances are more common than they are elsewhere in North America. That apart, it was landing through clouds, which can also disrupt the electrical field—and which may have an electrical field of their own that is far different from that on the ground. Maxey claims that moisture in the clouds conducts pos-ions down from the ionosphere at such an increased rate that they may distort the surrounding electrical field. Maxey has argued in articles published in aeronautical journals that the end result "could favor induced currents in man's central nervous system, especially the brain, at frequencies tending toward trance states." He claims that such a temporary trancelike state could affect pilots under the heavy stress of making instrument landings. Says Maxey: "Picture yourself up there making a pretty good approach when all of a sudden without any awareness at all it's like somebody dropped a mickey on you. But you don't know its a mickey because you can't smell it, you can't taste it, you can't feel it. The next thing you know—without any explanation—the runway's sitting right smack in front of you."

To support his theory Maxey points out that there was a time lapse between the flight recorder in Flight 401 "hearing" the danger signal and the pilots reacting to it. He also claims that the U.S. Air Force once commissioned a study that involved installing a device in plane cockpits that generated fields similar to those found over open land. Maxey says that pilots using this equipment were less fatigued and had faster reaction times than pilots operating under ordinary conditions.

In Germany, Daimler-Benz examined the effect of electrical force fields in closed cars at the same time that they studied ionization counts and balances. One conclusion was that in closed cars most drivers' reaction time slows down dramatically. During the Second World War the German Luftwaffe considered suggestions from scientists that pilot fatigue might be caused by either the pos-ion to neg-ion balance or by the "unnatural" electrical field generated within closed cockpits—or by both at once.

If any scientific work was done by the Germans at that time the results have been lost or destroyed. But it is important to remember that prior to the War most aircraft had open cockpits or flew so slowly that the pilot simply opened the window for ventilation. During the thirties, however, the Luftwaffe pioneered the use of faster, higher-flying bombers and fighters with enclosed cockpits whose windows could not be opened. The pilots were thus locked inside a man-made microenvironment, just as we so often are in cars.

Research into the effects of the earth's natural electrical field is so new that it will be years before most of today's theories can be either proved or disproved. But if it is finally demonstrated that the natural force field is crucial to human physical and mental well-being, then those of us who work and live in modern high-rise buildings are troubled by more than pos-ion poisoning. Those buildings—the newer ones at least—are built largely from manufactured materials; steel, reinforced cement, synthetic siding, and so on. As a result they almost amount to Faraday cages; that is, rooms used by scientists that are so well insulated with copper that no external electrical influences or radio waves can penetrate the walls. No apartment or office is that efficient a cage, but high-rise buildings do tend to exclude, or at least disturb, the natural electrical field that exists outside. They also tend to keep in the "alien" electrical fields created by appliances such as stoves, toasters, TV sets, electric typewriters, and copying machines. Older structures of traditional brick and stone are said to cause few, if any, problems, but Henry L. Logan, the New York engineer who believes that the newer artificial environments have "changed the rules of survival," has also pointed out that: "Until now, man has only had to contend with the natural fields to which he has adapted, but in this century Western man particularly is being exposed to increasingly distorted artificial electrical fields largely undetected by the senses, lacking therapeutic benefits of the natural fields, and harmful in many ways." Dr. Stark sounds even more alarming on the subject. He says that "Ionization is like the water in which a man swims. He would have no trouble in a natural environment, but because we have upset things he cannot swim well; just about stay afloat in fact. Artificial electrical fields may be the last straw. They are like waves that come along to make things worse, and if the waves are too high or too rough then our swimmer may be swamped."

In a Faraday cage, where the outside electrical fields are excluded, plants grow only about half the size they would if rooted in the garden. The human being isn't a philodendron or a geranium, but many people in apartment complexes complain that their plants are stunted or unhealthy or just won't grow, and sometimes I wonder whether that just might be true of people.

11

The Odyssey Continues

By the fall of 1972 my research odyssey had taken me far enough into the subject of the ion effect for me to believe it would be worthwhile setting up a clinic in Geneva similar to Felix Sulman's in Jerusalem. There were, I felt, two obvious benefits: It would help other Foehn victims, and be profitable as well. I tried and I failed, largely because before I could raise enough money, the doctor who was to be a partner was compelled to find other employment.

A year later the Swiss Meteorological Institute produced its formal report, "Foehn and Weather Sensitiveness," that not only confirmed all the hand-me-down stories about the Foehn being an ill wind, but also proved that much of what I had come to believe about the ion effect was in fact completely true. Perhaps my attempt to start a clinic for treatment of the Foehn disease was just a little before its time. The Meteorological Institute's confirmation that the Foehn was a Witches' Wind to be blamed for many of the ills that beset humankind in mountainous middle Europe might have made my clinic a far more attractive enterprise. Certainly the report was followed by the first of what were to be many newspaper articles on the evils of the Swiss climate in general and the Geneva situation in particular.

On the whole, the Swiss Meteorological Institute was tentative in its acknowledgment of the ion effect as a major factor in Foehn sickness. Paradoxically, it recommended the treatments devised by Felix Sulman in Jerusalem as one possible cure, but did not refer to the fact that Sulman is, in fact, treating cases of pos-ion poisoning. However, many ion scientists would regard even this lukewarm acceptance of the importance of ionization as a triumph of sorts. As recently as the late 1960s Albert Krueger wrote, "It is disconcerting at times to find that some of our peers classify the subject with the occult arts." The kind of scornful skepticism that prompted that statement no longer exists, but there is still a staggering amount of suspicion and disagreement among ion scientists themselves. Often scientists seem to totally disregard the ion effect—perhaps out of ignorance. For instance, in 1976 Dr. Otmar Harlfinger and Dr. Gerd Jendritzky of the Medical Meteorological Department of the West German Weather Station in Freiburg, published the results of a four-year study proving that industrial accidents are more frequent during the Foehn than at other times of the year. They also suggested that the Foehn might explain the sudden rise in the number of traffic accidents. But for all the studies and reports on the ion effect—and despite the fact that the Swiss Meteorological Institute had only two years earlier cited ions as one cause of Foehn sickness—the two German scientists said they were unable even to suggest any explanation why the Foehn should have such an effect.

The disagreement between scientists is classically typified in the public exchange between Dr. I. Andersen and Dr. Albert Krueger. At the International Biometeorological Conference in Holland in 1972, Dr. Andersen said that investigations into the effect of ions on complex biological systems "must be considered preposterous." Dr. Krueger replied in a subsequent scientific paper by saying, "I do not concur with Dr.

Andersen's statements," and produced a flood of evidence to prove his point. In the low-key, understated world of high science that is the equivalent of two politicians having a bitter row.

The skepticism is, however, diminishing. One major breakthrough came in 1972, when I contacted Dr. G. Lambert, then an environmental psychologist in the World Health Organization's occupational health department. Although he conceded that the W.H.O. was not then spending much on ion research, he did display interest in the research material I had amassed, and later wrote to me: "We are interested in the role played by ionization as a physical factor in the environment, in the health and behavior of man [and] I am particularly grateful for the help you are giving us." In 1975 the W.H.O. and the World Meteorological Association set up a joint study group on Higher Human Biometeorology—that is, the effects of weather and environments on humankind. It was, in fact, a belated response to worldwide concern about the way we are damaging our physical and mental health by creating, with pollution and artificial indoor climates, unhealthy mini- and micro-environments. In 1976 the two world organizations recommended that as "a matter of urgency" all nations study, among other things, "the possible action of various parameters of natural electricity on man."

Perhaps the scientific establishment may be forgiven its dilatory response to ion research since so much of it has been and is being done by poorly financed scientists working in isolation. What Dr. Davis of N.A.S.A.'s Andrews Air Force Base wrote in 1962 is still largely true: "Most work on ionized air effects has been performed by researchers working largely independent of each other. They have seldom met to discuss their respective work and plans. Even where a single body has sponsored the pursuit of any diverse research project in the field, there has been no really adequate central direction as far as the medical research program goes."

Even so, there is overwhelming evidence to prove

conclusively that in the past half century man has, with some good intent and considerable ignorance, meddled with the environment so much that the ion balance has been distorted and in places destroyed, so that the minds and bodies of almost all city and urban residents and workers are to some extent affected. You can't ride a bus, drive a car, or even buy a new suit or dress made of synthetics without being, in one way or another, a victim of the ion effect. The staggering reader response to that story in the *Ottawa Journal* in Canada shows that we are all conscious that *something* is amiss with our living and working environments.

The report of the initial conference of the W.H.O.–W.M.O. group on Higher Human Biometeorology, which was sent to all U.N. member nations, said, "It is agreed that cooperation with architects, engineers, and town planners should be improved to include relevant aspects of human biometeorology because housing conditions are very important, in particular for people no longer able to adapt [to urban environments]. Architects are very often inclined to pay more attention to the aesthetic and economical factors and hence to sacrifice the human biometeorological aspects. At the planning stage of preparing architectural designs, the factors associated with human well-being have to be taken into account as of primary importance."

It will be a long time before the last word can be written on the subject of the ion effect. But clearly there are both long-term and short-term solutions to the way we are currently damaging ourselves through ion depletion and pos-ion poisoning.

In buildings, ionizers able to generate "healthy" levels of both pos-ions and neg-ions can be installed. People are, as we have seen, already using ionizers effectively in many parts of the world, and they are healthier and happier because of them. In cars and all private vehicles you can use the small neg-ion generators to compensate for the overproduction of pos-ions. The problem is more complex in airplanes, but I infer from the report of F.A.A. researchers that the problem in airplanes is just as serious. More research would provide a solution. In homes and offices where there is no central air-conditioning system to which ion generators could be linked, you can use either room- or office-sized ionizers that are far less costly and complex than, say, a wall or window air conditioner or electric heater.

While no one would suggest that we know all there is to know about the ion effect, there is the evidence of a quarter century of research throughout the world that proves one thing conclusively: *There is no harmful consequence from the artificial generation of neg-ions except, perhaps, that they may keep you alert and awake for longer than you need be.* There is no apparent reason why, even before more research is undertaken, we should not straighten out the ion imbalance in offices, apartments, schools, houses, factories, and other places where we live and work by using neg-ion generators.

At the present state of the technology, however, these are stopgap measures. A great deal more research is needed both to refine the existing types of ion generators and ion counters, and to determine what is the best ion level to maintain. In the past some ionizers have been ineffective, but it is in the area of dosages that most work needs to be done, particularly when using ions as a medical treatment or therapy. The number of ions in the air in natural conditions can vary without apparent effect on human beings; for instance, the total number of ions can reach 100,000 per cubic centimeter—as in the massive overdose of neg-ions near a waterfall such as Niagara Falls—and drop to the "natural" level of around 1,000 to 2,000 total ions just a quarter mile away. The Russians say that when they give neg-ion medical treatments lasting between 15 and 30 minutes, a dosage of 10 million neg-ions produces the same effect as one of 100 million. The evidence suggests that ion depletion and pos-ion overdoses produce the most damaging effects; massive quantities of ions where the pos-ion to neg-ion ratio is normal or massive overdoses of neg-ions don't hurt. Rather, they are generally beneficial, though Danish researcher Christian Bach points out that spending too long in a neg-ion enriched environment might keep you alert and awake and result in a lack of rest if the dosage is too high. There is less disagreement about pos-ion overdoses: The scientific literature contains a report of one study where scientists put 40 volunteers into a room containing 32 million pos-ions per cubic centimeter. All got sick within minutes, and some had to be carried out.

The Russians market a make-it-yourself neg-ion generator kit and it became so popular that in 1972 the authorities issued an official warning that if you don't actually need to use it you are in danger of keeping yourself too alert and active to sleep. Neg-ion generators are manufactured in North America, but the regulations of the U.S. and Canada forbid them to be promoted as anything but "air cleaners." In the U.S. ionizers may be used for experimental purposes in universities and private laboratories, but the Food and Drug Administration refuses to permit them to be sold to the public (and some caution on their part is both understandable and commendable). The F.D.A. is saying: "Prove to us, by standards U.S. science accepts, that not only do these devices ionize the air adequately, but that they do have the therapeutic effects claimed." Private interests are trying to do just that. One U.S. firm is helping finance research projects at U.S. universities and institutional laboratories.

But it's very little, very late. Ion depletion and pos-ion poisoning are at least as harmful to the environment and to human beings as any known form of pollution. Yet governments take action on pollution, both in financing research and in passing antipollution legislation, while so far as I can find out no public money has been spent on ion science beyond a few thousand dollars in grants to Albert Krueger at the University of California. Currently, he is being financed by the U.S. Navy to study the effect of low-energy force fields on small animals. The world's most authoritative scientist in what appears to be an area of research of massive significance in the late twentieth century is currently financed by the Pentagon to the tune of a $45,000 grant, and is obliged to carry on the work for which he is internationally renowned in his spare time.

In fairness, Dr. Krueger says he was well financed by government agencies until 1970, when all research funds began to dry up. But the fact that he is now allotted no more than it would cost to open a hamburger franchise suggests to me that our value system is at least somewhat distorted, if not downright crazy. Dr. Krueger himself is disappointed that the government-backed scientific establishment hasn't taken a more active interest in extending his basic research. Publicly, however, all he says is, "It appears air ion investigations constitute a legitimate and even promising branch of biological research." Federal authorities must recognize that the ion effect is the challenge of the 1970s, just as pollution was the challenge, still to be met, of the 1960s. They should realize that the U.S. lags behind other developed nations where ionization is concerned. There should be enough money available for ion scientists to do the research that is desperately needed. The ion scientists I met on my odyssey of research are all eager for this to happen. They say that once the wealth and energy of the U.S. is thrown behind ion science, all, or at least most, of the questions that remain will soon be answered. As I hope I have demonstrated, it is vital to the health of the human race that these questions be answered, and quickly.

The F.A.A. researchers who studied the ion effect after air traffic controllers complained about pos-ion concentrations in radar rooms concluded that, "The atmosphere is our most precious natural resource. Since we all breathe air from the day we are born until the day we die, and since atmospheric ions have been shown to exert significant effects on living organisms, the fact that there is relatively little on-going research concerning their physical nature and behavioral, psychological, and biochemical effects seems appalling."

Antipollution laws, particularly those governing

motor vehicle exhaust emissions, will help alleviate some of the ion-depletion problems in cities and urban areas. In time, air conditioning and central heating systems will by law be designed so that their effect on the ion count and balance will be minimal, and ion generators will be built as part of heating and cooling systems. We will also almost certainly reach the point where all building materials will be approved only if they are not likely to upset the ion effect. And I expect that all furnishings and clothing made with synthetic fibers will have either their positive or negative potential listed along with the washing and cleaning instructions. Better still, there may be legislation demanding that these synthetics be treated chemically to neutralize their electrostatic potential entirely. But reaching the point where these things come about will require more and massive research to convince the F.D.A. and other regulatory bodies. And that research —as the World Health Organization has already decided—should be started now "as a matter of urgency." We ion sensitives can't wait, and we are a quarter of the population. And, as the Ottawa experience shows, we are not the only ones who suffer. Everybody does.

I myself feel infinitely better since I left Geneva and moved back to North America. The decision to leave Geneva was a hard one to make. For me, that city was both paradise and purgatory—and when I was not suffering from my Geneva condition, the paradise element was overwhelmingly seductive. In retrospect, the report on Foehn sickness by the Swiss Meteorological Institute sums up the reasons why, in 1974, I finally wrenched myself away and took a job in Canada.

In addition to discussing the effects of various drugs and ionizers on the problem, Gian Gensler, the author of the Swiss report, also said that those people with sensitive nervous systems most readily affected by the Foehn should recognize that as they enter their thirties their systems are less able to withstand stress, and the pressures of work and of the ion effect can become intolerable. He suggested that such people adopt a "sensible" lifestyle as they age and exercise moderation in business as well as in eating and drinking habits. "Finally, not only the vegetative nervous system but the whole human being must be regenerated and taken care of as a psychosomatic unity—body and soul together," he wrote.

Well, by 1973 I was 42. I was taking serotonin blockers and using a neg-ion generator and was exercising moderation in all things—or at least most of them. In the years before I discovered the ion effect I had taken so many tranquilizers, stimulants, sleeping pills, and other medications to alleviate the medical symptoms of what I now know to be pos-ion poisoning, that my body chemistry was more out of balance than it had ever been. But none of the suggested cures worked—I was still suffering. And so I took the final piece of advice implicit in all the Institute's findings: I moved.

I am still more sensitive than most to the ion effect. Like most people, businessmen and women particularly, I am forced to spend a large part of my life in high-rise buildings; indeed, the job I returned to North America to do involved my having an office on the fifty-second floor of a Toronto skyscraper. I still find that after spending hours in such a building my energy level falls below par, and I may have a sudden mood change or feel strangely weary and apathetic— all afflictions suffered by many of my colleagues and friends who must endure similar environments at work and at home. But I have one advantage—I *know* what's wrong, and most of them don't. When you are depressed or anxious and can't explain why, you breed more depression and anxiety because you fear the unknown cause. And I no longer have to fear the unknown—when I feel out of sorts I now know I am probably suffering from a dose of pos-ion poisoning. Perhaps this book will help you conquer your fear of this unknown.

By all that's sane and reasonable, the weight of scientific evidence demonstrating that the ion effect is damaging to everybody is now so great that governments must do something, and soon, to ease or even end the cause of the distress that I and so many others have felt. The governments have shown precious little inclination to do anything so far, and this book is an attempt to prod them into action. You, the reader, can help, because if you're not worried now, then you should be.

Chapter 16: Question

Selected Bibliography

Becker, Robert O., M.D. "Electromagnetic Forces and
  Life Forces." *Technology Review*. Cambridge: Massa-
  chusetts Institute of Technology, 1972.
Beckman, Harry L., M.D. "Negatively Charged Atomic
  Oxygen and Its Impact on Biology and Pathology of
  Life Processes." Naples, Italy: Proceedings of the Fifth
  International Congress of Cybernetic Medicine, 1968.
Blain, Barry. "Negative Ions: In the Air?" Police Scien-
  tific Development Branch, Technical Memorandum.
  U.K. Government Home Office, 1974.
Burgess, Howard F. "Strange Power of Air Ions." *Popular
  Electronics*, 1969.
Cone, Clarence D., Jr. "Control of Cell Division by the
  Electrical Voltage of the Surface Membrane." San
  Antonio, Texas: Proceedings of the Twelfth Annual
  Science Writers' Seminar of the American Cancer
  Society, March, 1970.
Elasser, Walter M. "The Earth as a Dynamo." *Scientific
  American*, May, 1958.
Flying Magazine. Special Instrument Flying Issue, 1973.
Friedman, Howard. "Geomagnetic Parameters and Psy-
  chiatric Hospital Admissions. Syracuse Veterans Ad-
  ministration Hospital, et al." *Nature Magazine*, 1963.
Gaultierotti, R.; Kornblueh, I. H.; and Sitori, C., eds.
  Bioclimatology, Biometeorology and Aeroionotherapy,
  Milan: Carlo Erba Foundation, 1968.

————. *Aeroionotherapy*. Milan: Carlo Erba Foundation, 1968.

Gensler, Gian. *Klimatologie Der Schweiz, Part II*. Zurich: Die Schweizerische Meterologische Zentralanstalt, 1973.

Graeffe, Gunnar, et al. *The Ions in the Air in the Sauna*. Finland: Department of Physics, Tempere University of Technology, 1974.

Kerdo, I., M.D.; Hay, Gy; and Svab, F. *New Possibilities in the Increasing of Driving Safety*. Budapest, Hungary: Medicor, 1973.

Kimura, Schoichi, et al. "Influence of the Air Lacking in Light Ions and the Effect of Its Artificial Ionization upon Human Beings in Occupied Rooms." Japan: Imperial University, August, 1938.

Kornblueh, Igho, M.D., et al. "Polarized Air as an Adjunct in the Treatment of Burns." Philadelphia: Northeastern Hospital, 1959.

Krueger, A. P. "The Action of Air Ions on Bacteria." *Journal of General Physiology*. Berkeley: University of California, 1957.

————. "Effects of Air Ions on Trachea of Primates." Proceedings of the Society of Experimental Biological Medicine, U.S.A., 1959.

————. "The Biological Mechanisms of Air Ion Action." *Journal of General Physiology*. Berkeley: University of California, 1957.

————. "The Biological Properties of Gaseous Ions." *The Encyclopedia of Science and Technology*. New York: McGraw-Hill, 1962.

————. "Influences of Air Ions on Certain Physiological Functions." *Medical Biometeorology—Weather Climate and the Living Organism*. Amsterdam, London and New York: Elsevier, 1963.

————. "Air Ion Effects on the Iron Metabolism of Barley." Japan: Proceedings of the Botanical Society, 1965.

————. "Small Air Ions: Their effect on blood levels of serotonin in terms of modern physical theory." *International Journal of Biometeorology*, Vol. 12, 1968.

————. "Are Air Ions Biologically Significant?"—A Review of a Controversial Subject." *International Journal of Biometeorology*, 1972.

————. "Are Negative Air Ions Good For You?" *The New Scientist*. United Kingdom, June 14, 1973.

————. "The Influence of Air Ions on a Model of Respiratory Disease." Paris: Proceedings of the World Congress of Medicine and Biology of the Environment, 1974.

Laws, C. A., and Holiday, E. R. "Air Ions in Physical Medicine and Environmental Hygiene." Proceedings of the Symposium of the British Society of Environmental Engineers, 1975.

Logan, Henry L. "Light and the Human Environment." *Journal of the World Institute Council,* U.S.A., Summer, 1974.

Minkh, A. A., "The Effect of Ionized Air on Work Capacity and Vitamin Metabolism." *Journal of the Academy of Medical Sciences, U.S.S.R.* Translated by U.S. Department of Commerce, Washington, D.C., 1961.

————. "Aero-Ionization in Medicine." *Journal of the Academy of Medical Sciences, U.S.S.R.* Translation distributed by the Office of Technical Services, U.S. Department of Commerce, Washington D.C., 1961.

Mishlove, Jeffrey. *The Roots of Consciousness.* New York: Random House, 1975.

Rosenberg, Bruce L. "A Study of Atmospheric Ionization." Atlantic City, New Jersey: National Aviation Facilities Experimental Center, May 1972.

Selby, Miriam and Earl. "Beware the Witch's Wind." *National Wildlife Magazine,* August-September, 1972.

Sharp, E. L. *Relation of Air Ions to Air Pollution and Some Biological Effects.* U.K.: Applied Science Publishers Ltd., 1972.

Silverman, Daniel, M.D. et al. "Effect of Artificial Ionization of the Air on the Electroencephalogram." *American Journal of Physical Medicine,* 1957.

Stark, Walter. *Vitaionen—ein potentieller Gesundheitsfaktor.* Lugano, Switzerland: Tipografia, 1971.

————. *Die Bibel Weist Modernster Wissenschaft den Weg.* Geneva: Ariston Verlag, 1975.

Sulfsohn, Norman L., ed. "The Nervous System and Electric Currents." Las Vegas, Nevada: Proceedings of the Third Annual National Conference of the Neuro-Electric Society, 1970.

Sulman, F. G. "Effects of Hot Dry Desert Winds (Sharav, Hamsin) on the Metabolism of Hormones." *Journal of the Medical Association of Israel,* 1962.

————. "Urinalysis of Patients Suffering from Climatic

Heat Stress (Sharav)." *International Journal of Biometeorology*, vol. 14, 1970.

————. "Serotonin-Migraine in Climatic Heat Stress, Its Prophylaxis and Treatment." Elsinore, Denmark: Proceedings of the International Headache Symposium, 1971.

————. "The Role of Serotonin in Gynaecology and Obstetrics." *The Hebrew Pharmacist*, vol. 14.

————. "Adrenal Medullary Exhaustion from Tropical Winds and Its Management." *Israel Journal of Medical Sciences*, 1973.

————. "Meteorological Front Movements and Human Weather Sensitivity." Karger Gazette, 1974.

————. "Air-Ionometry of Hot, Dry Desert Winds (Sharav) and Treatment with Air Ions of Weather-Sensitive Subjects." *International Journal of Biometeorology*, vol. 18, 1974.

————. "Climatic Factors in the Incidence of Attacks of Migraine." *Hemicrania Journal of the Migraine Trust of Great Britain*, 1974.

————. "Influence of Artificial Air Ionisation on the Human Electroencephalogram." *International Journal of Biometeorology*, vol. 18, 1974.

Tchijewsky, A. L. "Air Ionization, Its Role in the National Economy." Moscow: State Planning Commission of the U.S.S.R. Translated by the Office of Naval Intelligence, Washington, D.C., 1960.

Tromp, S. W., ed. "Progress in Human Biometeorology." Amsterdam: Swets and Zeitlinger, 1974.

University of Maryland. Proceedings of the Seventh International Biometeorological Congress, 1975.

Wehner, Alfred. P. "Electro-aerosol Therapy." *American Journal of Physical Medicine*, vol. 41, 1962.

Wever, R. "Human Cicadian Rhythms Under the Influence of Weak Electric Fields and the Different Aspects of These Studies." *International Journal of Biometeorology*, vol. 17, 1973.

World Meteorological Organization. "Applications of Meteorology and Climatology to the Biosphere and the Human Environment." Geneva: Proceedings of the Commission for Special Applications of Meteorology and Climatology, 1973.

————. "A Survey of Human Biometeorology," Technical Note No. 65, 1974.

Index

abortion, 126–27
acupuncture, 52
Acute Migrannus Neuralgia, 76, 113
Adam, Gygorgy, 110
adrenaline, 29–30, 39, 41, 56
Aeroinotherapy Journal, 126
aerosol therapy, 70–72
air conditioning, *see* central heating and air conditioning
Air Ionization: Its Role in the National Economy (Tchijewsky), 56
airplanes:
  accidents, 14, 100–1, 113, 114–15, 137–38
  atmospheric conditions in, 112–15, 137–38
alcohol, 7
  overindulgence in, 10, 103, 113
allergies:
  respiratory problems caused by, 70, 73, 82
Alpha waves, 45
American Journal of Physical Medicine, 71
Andersen, Dr. I., 141–42
Andrews, Dr. Edson, 60
animal behavior:
  moving weather fronts and, 22–23

animals:
  ionization experiments and, 20, 33–34, 40, 43–45, 52, 77, 90, 110, 125–26, 145
antibiotics, 64
anxiety, 2, 4, 6, 10, 13, 23, 29, 34, 38, 41, 91
  neg-ion overdoses for, 44–45, 103
  serotonin and, 76
  among urban dwellers, 46, 102–4
anxiolytics, 7, 103
appliances, electrical:
  artificially generated electrical field of, 130, 139
Arabs, 136
  Sharav and, 36, 41
architects, human biometeorology and, 143
asthma, 32, 40, 68, 69, 72, 78
  babies with, 57
  humidity and, 82
  statistics on, 70
  synthetics and, 117, 118–20
athletes, experimentation with, 53–56
Austria:
  Foehn wind and, 17, 23, 89, 107, 135
  suicide rate in, 135
automatic nervous system, 78
  pos-ions for underactive, 48

ABOUT THE AUTHORS

FRED SOYKA is a Canadian business executive and graduate engineer who spent twelve years in Geneva, Switzerland, a city plagued by "Witches' Winds." They made his life, like those of many Geneva residents, unbearable. Seeking a reason why, he set out on an odyssey of discovery that led him to amass a unique body of material on the subject of ions and how they affect us all.

ALAN EDMONDS is one of North America's most seasoned journalists. He was for years correspondent for the London *Daily Express* and for the Toronto *Daily Star,* and then a writer and editor for *Maclean's* and *The Canadian Magazine.* He is the author of *Voyage to the Edge of the World.*

How's Your Health?

Bantam publishes a line of informative books, written by top experts to help you toward a healthier and happier life.

Bantam Book Catalog

Here's your up-to-the-minute listing of over 1,400 titles by your favorite authors.

This illustrated, large format catalog gives a description of each title. For your convenience, it is divided into categories in fiction and non-fiction—gothics, science fiction, westerns, mysteries, cookbooks, mysticism and occult, biographies, history, family living, health, psychology, art.

So don't delay—take advantage of this special opportunity to increase your reading pleasure.

Just send us your name and address and 50¢ (to help defray postage and handling costs).